Objective Structured Clinical Examination
for Psychiatric Trainees
volume II

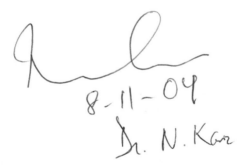

8-11-04

Dr. N. Kar

Also available from Quay Books, MA Healthcare Limited:

Objective Structured Clinical Examintion for Psychiatric Trainees, volume I by Jaap van der Boom, Joseph Tony and Srinivasa Thirumalai
Vignettes for the MRCPsych, second edition by Robert Cohen
Presentations of Clinical Psychiatry by Robert Cohen

Objective Structured Clinical Examination for Psychiatric Trainees
volume II

Jaap van der Boom, Joseph Tony, Srinivasa Thirumalai

Quay Books
MA Healthcare Limited

Quay Books Division, MA Healthcare Limited, Jesses Farm, Snow Hill, Dinton, Salisbury, Wiltshire, SP3 5HN

British Library Cataloguing-in-Publication Data
A catalogue record is available for this book

© MA Healthcare Limited 2004
ISBN 1 85642 275 5

Printed in the UK by Cromwell Press, Trowbridge

Contents

Section three: Communication skills

Foreword

With the introduction of the Objective Structured Clinical Examination (OSCE), the Royal College of Psychiatrists has taken another step to ensure that its examination tests how well candidates treat patients.

In medicine, it is no good knowing what is in the textbooks if you do not know how to apply that knowledge for the benefit of your patients on the wards, in the clinic and in the community. The College has introduced the OSCE to test how candidates function as specialist psychiatric doctors.

In volume I, Drs Jaap van der Book, Joseph Tony and Srinivasa Thirumalai provided MRCPsych candidates with an admirable structure to help them prepare for the OSCE part of the examination.

A good clinician draws not only from textbook knowledge, but from experience of different clinical situations. In volume II, the authors build on the success of their first volume, keeping to the same useful and highly effective format. They provide here a further forty-five common clinical scenarios, helping you add breadth and depth to your knowledge of psychiatry and also making it most unlikely that even the most diligent candidate will run out of practice materials. Preparing for a major exam is never easy, but having a useful guide can smooth the path. For those preparing for the OSCE, you need look no further than the two volumes of this excellent series.

Good luck!

Robert Cohen
March, 2004

Introduction

This book is intended for those trainees preparing for the MRCPsych Part 1 examination. Objective structured clinical examinations (OSCEs) are being used to test a broad range of subjects and skills in a quantifiable and valid form.

The OSCE format was first used in the spring of 2003.

An OSCE differs from the traditional 'long case' exam, by using simulated cases or patients. The aim of this design is to reduce the likelihood of candidates having varying experiences with the same patient. OSCEs are designed to ensure that a range of skills are tested, with scores being allocated against clear and explicit criteria. They are more objective because each candidate is observed and assessed in a similar situation.

In the OSCEs, the roles are played by actors or in certain stations an anatomical model will be used. In that way a wide range of skills can be tested without having to recruit actual patients with specific symptoms or illnesses. Anatomical models allow skills to be tested that would normally be difficult to be conduct on actors or volunteers, eg. cardio-pulmonary resuscitation.

Candidates usually rotate around twelve OSCE stations, which last for seven minutes. The candidates all start at different station and then rotate around, completing the remaining stations. A bell is rung one minute before the seven minutes are over. There may be one or two rest stations.

Each OSCE station is designed to assess a particular skill within the core curriculum. The list of skills to be tested includes:

- eliciting a relevant history
- making a diagnosis
- clinical examination
- discussion of treatment options
- obtaining consent for treatment or procedures
- performing specific procedures
- discussion of test results and prognosis
- prescribing appropriate treatment.

How to use this book

This book contains a series of OSCE examples. The main chapters divide the OSCEs into those that focus on history-taking, communication, procedural and specific examination skills. Within each chapter are instructions for candidates, actors and examiners. The instructions for examiners include marking criteria and sample answers. The answers that we have written are only a rough guide to what you might say or do in the actual exam. With practice, you will hopefully be able to improve on our answers and develop your own personal style, with which you feel comfortable.

We would suggest that, if possible, you try to practice by doing role play in a small group. One person could take the role of the candidate, another could be the actor and the others could act as examiners. It is also important that somebody keeps a track of the time. Try to stick to the time frame of seven minutes and the warning with forty seconds to go, so that you get a feel for it. Candidates are given a minute to read the instructions and gather their thoughts. The actors may need some more time to get into their role.

For the role of examiner we have given some suggestions about the way the OSCEs can be approached. This is, however, not the only correct way. It is important that you come up with an approach that shows understanding and insight. We have also added some ratings which can be used by the examiners. We would suggest you go over the OSCE afterwards, to see in which areas you have done well and where you could still improve. You will benefit most from these sessions when you use positive feedback.

If you can, get an SpR or a Consultant involved.

For the 'procedural' OSCEs we have provided relevant check lists as physical examination does not easily lend itself to being assessed in a textbook. 'Procedural' OSCEs might also be best done in groups.

How are OSCEs marked?

This page shows a specimen check-list for an OSCE station. You will notice the different and very specific attributes of a candidate that are examined.

	Excellent A	Good B	Average C	Fail D	Severe fail E
Introduction					
Rapport					
Consent					
Listening skills					
Verbal facilitation					
Question framing					
Emotional content					
Explanation					
Diagnostic criteria					
Factual knowledge					
Summarization					
Patient's concerns and perceptions					
Ending					

Table Introduction.1: Check-list for an OSCE station

Preparing for the examination

⌘ It is useful, and makes sense to practice OSCEs in groups.
⌘ Make a list of likely OSCEs, dividing them according to skills tested or even disorders.
⌘ Ask for practice sessions with local SpRs or Consultant trainers, who have an interest in the field.
⌘ Practice often, though how often is up to you! We have found that it is useful to repeat OSCEs after an interval of up to several days, to see whether there is an actual improvement in your scores.
⌘ Practice all the roles so that you not only get to know what it's like on the 'other' side, but also get an idea of what really works or impresses.
⌘ Try to stick to exam conditions — the pressure can be intense!

Tips for success on the day

⌘ Arrive early and look your best. Make sure you have slept enough the previous night!
⌘ Introduce yourself to the patient and outline what you are going to do in broad terms.
⌘ Listen to the patient. You might have a task to do, but you are also being observed on the details of your interaction with the patient.
⌘ Pick-up clues in what the patient says to you. They might give you openings or ways out of difficult situations.
⌘ Adapt to the situation. Although we have tried to cover as many potential areas as we could, be prepared for anything.
⌘ Stop yourself from asking questions as if from a list. Practice different types of questions including open-ended questions ('Tell me about…') that allow the patient to expand on his/her answers.
⌘ Be sensitive to the situation and the patient.
⌘ Obtain consent for any procedure.
⌘ Explain everything!
⌘ Watch your technique – don't be careless in disposing of used medical instruments.

Remember that there are many stations, so you have more than just one opportunity to show that you measure up to the standard. Even if you remember a vital point/question some way into the question, try to incorporate it into what you are doing. You can't be failed for correcting a mistake.

What are the examiners looking for?

⌘ Confidence.
⌘ Good communication.
⌘ Flexibility in questioning style.

⌘ Reasonable factual knowledge.
⌘ Competence in performing procedures.
⌘ Balanced approach.
⌘ Demonstrates empathy.
⌘ Treats the station as if it were 'real' life.
⌘ Being sensitive to a patient's distress or anxiety.
⌘ Demonstrates reasonable control of interview.

We hope that by using these OSCEs to revise your skills, you will be better prepared to face the actual examination.

Good Luck!

Jaap van der Boom
Joseph Tony
Srinivasa Thirumalai

March, 2004

Section one:
History-taking skills

Instructions for candidates

1. Nightmares and night terrors

A GP has referred this twenty-four-year-old lady to your outpatient clinic after concerns about her sleep pattern. She had been found the previous night by her boyfriend, wandering around the bedroom with a paperweight in her hands. She has no recollection of the incident but is obviously distressed.

Elicit the relevant history.

2. Erectile dysfunction

This twenty-nine-year-old man has been referred by his GP for an assessment of sexual dysfunction.

Assess his presenting complaints.

3. Forensic history

This twenty-four-year-old man is an inpatient on your ward. He was admitted after taking an overdose of heroin. Your consultant would like you to find out more about his contact with the criminal justice system.

Elicit his forensic history.

4. Confusion and visual hallucinations

Mr Jones lives with his seventy-eight-year-old wife. She was admitted to the old age psychiatry ward last night after she was found wandering in the corridor of their sheltered accommodation. She had unrolled the fire-hose to chase away wild animals that she claimed she could see.

Elicit a collateral history.

5. Depression with psychotic symptoms

You have been asked to see this seventy-eight-year-old widow. She had a mild stroke six months ago, from which she has made a good recovery. For the last three months however she has become increasingly depressed. She has become quite preoccupied with certain ideas which worry her greatly.

Assess her presenting complaints, and any unusual beliefs that she may have.

6. Excessive day-time sleepiness

You have been asked to see this forty-five-year-old man by his GP. His main complaint is of excessive sleepiness during the day. He wants help for the problem.

Elicit the relevant history and give advice as necessary.

7. Chronic pain

This is a forty-year-old mathematics teacher, with an eight-year history of abdominal pain. He has had a range of tests and investigations, but no cause for the pain has been found. His GP suggested that he see a psychiatrist, to which he has reluctantly agreed.

Elicit relevant history, paying special attention to emotional and psycho-social factors that may play a role in his presentation.

8. History of an epileptic seizure

Nursing staff on a psychiatric ward have asked you to review this thirty-four-year old lady who was admitted three days ago for a relapse of her psychotic illness. She appears to have had an epileptic fit. The nursing staff say that she suddenly fell to the ground and had what looked like a grand-mal seizure. After having been unresponsive for about five minutes the patient has now recovered.

Elicit a relevant history and possible precipitating factors.

9. Substance-induced psychosis

You are asked to see this twenty-eight-year-old man from Somalia. He has been referred to you by his GP because he complains of persecutory ideas and auditory hallucinations.

Elicit a relevant history.

10. Social phobia

A twenty-seven-year-old man, who works as a middle grade manager has come to see you. He is a bachelor and lives alone. He had been to see his GP for a sick note. He said that he didn't feel that he could attend meetings with his colleagues or have meals with them. He was scared he would say the wrong thing or embarrass himself in front of them.

Assess his symptoms.

11. Chronic fatigue syndrome

This thirty-five-year-old lady, who last worked as a secretary one year ago, has been referred to your outpatient clinic by her GP. She has had numerous investigations for her complaints of chronic fatigue and joint and muscle pains, and the GP now feels that she needs a psychiatric assessment.

Clarify the presenting complaints and assess for symptoms of chronic fatigue syndrome.

12. Morbid jealousy

A forty-year-old married man, who works at a grocery, has come to see you. He has seen his GP to ask for antidepressant medication because he is convinced that his wife is being unfaithful to him. He has been drinking more alcohol than usual in the last few months.

Assess his symptoms.

13. Hypochondriasis

This forty-year-old man has been referred by his GP, who has performed numerous investigations for his occasional headaches and has not found any serious cause. The patient is convinced that he has a brain tumour. He has not responded to reassurance even after being seen by a neurologist, and constantly seeks more investigations. He spends most of his time at home collecting information on the internet about brain tumours. The GP thinks that he may be a hypochondriac.

Elicit relevant history and confirm the provisional diagnosis.

14. Postnatal depression

This thirty-five-year-old lady has been referred to your outpatient clinic because her GP is worried that she has become depressed after the birth of her first child four months ago. She is currently on maternity leave from her work as a postmistress. She has talked to her husband about feeling very low in mood and about having suicidal thoughts at times. She has also fought the impulse to throw her child out of the window of their second storey flat. Her husband is a teacher and has taken the last week off from work as he is concerned at his wife's state of mind and is also worried for his child's safety. They have both attended today's appointment.

Clarify the presenting complaints and assess for postnatal depression.

1.2

Instructions for actors

1. Nightmares and night terrors

You are a twenty-four-year-old female university student. You have a part-time shop assistant's job. You tend to drink and smoke at weekends. You have been with your current boyfriend for six years, and have a good relationship with your parents and younger sister.

Over the last year your sleep has become gradually more disrupted. You have been waking up in the middle of the night, screaming out aloud, sweating and feeling your heart racing. You don't know why you've been waking up, and can't recall any bad dreams or nightmares. Otherwise, there are no other problems with your everyday memory, and you are mentally well.

You went to see your doctor because, last night, your boyfriend found you walking with your eyes closed and a paperweight in your hands. He was able to wake you up and you were able to get back to sleep in bed. You have had similar episodes, occurring at least three times a week over the last few months. They usually happen in the early part of the night, less than an hour after you go off to sleep. On one occasion, you even slapped your boyfriend when he tried to wake you up. Last night's episode, has made you feel a bit more worried, as you might have accidentally hurt someone seriously. This morning, when discussing it with your family, you found out that your mother used to sleepwalk, and that you used to wet the bed until you were almost twelve.

2. Erectile dysfunction

You are a twenty-nine-year-old father of two, married for the last eleven years. You smoke twenty cigarettes a day and drink alcohol mostly at weekends. There is a family history of diabetes. You have had one previous episode of depression four years ago, and are being treated for your current episode with an antidepressant called paroxetine. At the moment, your mood is back to normal. Your main problem is that you have been unable to have an erection, when getting ready to have sexual intercourse, for at least a month. However, you are able to have erections early in the morning without being sexually aroused. Your wife has been very understanding and supportive. Despite this, you are worried that this problem will adversely affect your relationship. You have asked your GP for help, and he has referred you to a psychiatrist.

3. Forensic history

You are a twenty-four-year-old single man, admitted to hospital after taking an accidental overdose of heroin. You have just completed a twelve-month community rehabilitation order (CRO) after your fifth arrest for supplying class 'A' illicit drugs. You have been to prison on the four previous occasions.

You have been in and out of young offenders institutions since the age of seventeen. Your initial offences were of an acquisitive nature, mostly shoplifting (six convictions), and driving off without paying for petrol (bilking). On one occasion, you were caught setting fire to a shed. You had previously set fire to bins whilst truanting off school. Other, more recent offences over the last two years include actual bodily harm, assault, driving whilst being disqualified, and a few cautions for being drunk and disorderly.

4. Confusion and visual hallucinations

You are Mr Jones, an eighty-year-old man, who lives with his seventy-eight-year-old wife in sheltered accommodation. She was admitted to the old age psychiatry ward last night. This doctor wants to talk to you to get some more information about how things have been.

Your wife has been having brief spells of confusion on and off for the last year or so. These episodes can occur up to several times a day and can last for several hours at a time. During such an episode she does not seem to be quite herself. She is not sure about what time it is, or the day, and looks puzzled. You have heard her talking to children and animals that aren't there. With time, it has become increasingly difficult to reassure her and you have become quite worried. When she was found in a confused and agitated state last night, chasing imaginary animals with a fire hose, you realised that she was not safe to be at home anymore and agreed for her to be admitted to hospital.

She is not on any medication and has never been physically unwell. She has been walking with smaller, shuffling steps lately, and has fallen to the ground several times. The only other things you have noticed are that her face is not as animated as before and that she has had a slight tremor in her hands at times. You have had a difficult time looking after her in the last few months and it has been emotionally draining. When you talk about your story, you are tearful at times.

5. Depression with psychotic symptoms

You are a seventy-eight-year old lady whose husband died five years ago. Your middle aged sons live several hours away from you. You had a mild stroke six months ago, from which you made a good physical recovery. Initially you coped well, but in the last three months you have become increasingly low in mood. You have not attended to your self-care and have neglected house-hold chores. You find it very difficult to sleep at night and have been staying in bed during the day. Your appetite is poor and over the last three months your weight has dropped by around two stone. You have stopped going to church, and have given up working as treasurer for a fundraising initiative for orphans of AIDS in Africa. You are worried that the finances you controlled are in a mess and that everyone in church is blaming you for this. You have these thoughts on your mind constantly and are absorbed by guilt. You have been visited by fellow church-goers, who have tried to reassure you that there never has been a problem, but this has not helped.

You are also worried about your health. For the last few months, you have had some discharge 'down below' and noticed a bad smell. You are convinced that people are avoiding you because of this. You think that there may be something seriously wrong. These worries have been unbearable at times and you have thought about ending your life, but have not made any plans.

During the interview you are restless, and constantly wring your hands.

6. Excessive day-time sleepiness

You are an overweight, married forty-five-year-old man, with three children. You work for a printing company. For the last few years you have been feeling drowsy during the day. There have been times when, to your embarrassment, you have fallen asleep at work. You have also found yourself dozing off while driving your car, and have had to react quickly to avoid accidents.

You are generally fit and well, but feel that at eighteen stone, you are overweight. You aren't on any medication, but like to have a glass of whiskey as a nightcap.

You don't remember waking up at night, but your wife says that you snore loudly. She has also noticed that you sometimes stop breathing for a while and only start again after a loud snore.

You wonder why you feel sleepy all the time and would like to know whether there is anything that can be done about it.

7. Chronic pain

You are a forty-year-old married mathematics teacher with two grown up sons. Eight years ago you underwent a successful operation to repair a hernia in your groin. In the months following the operation you developed severe cramping pain, mainly in your lower abdomen. You have suffered with this pain ever since. You tend to feel bloated after a meal, and suffer from frequent bouts of diarrhoea, with the stool often mixed with mucus.

Milk, caffeine, alcohol and fatty foods tend to make the pain worse. Your persistent complaining has also put a strain on your marital relationship. The pain makes it hard for you to help with housework. Your wife doesn't understand what you are going through and often nags you, which makes you feel worse. You have also found that stress at work has a negative effect on the pain. You have been told that you suffer from irritable bowel syndrome (IBS) but are worried that there is something seriously wrong. Your father died ten years ago of bowel cancer. Over the years you have had several investigations including a range of blood-tests, a barium enema and colonoscopy. No abnormalities were found, but you are still not reassured and now put your hopes on a body scan. You have tried several medicines including pain killers and sedatives, but nothing has made a difference.

8. History of an epileptic seizure

You are a thirty-four-year-old woman, who has been unemployed for a year. You were admitted to the psychiatric ward three days ago, after hearing people talking about you when you were alone at home.

The nurses told you that you have just had an epileptic fit on the ward, but don't remember anything about it. You have a headache and your tongue feels as if you bit it.

You are confused, but are able to answer questions appropriately. Since coming to hospital you have had a few doses of a drug, but are not sure about the name.

Until your admission to hospital, you used to have alcohol binges and were taking at least three Valium tablets a day, which you bought off the street.

You have never had a fit before.

Please follow any instructions given to you by the candidate.

9. Substance-induced psychosis

You are a twenty-eight-year-old single man from Somalia. You came to the United Kingdom (UK) ten years ago. You are unemployed and spend a lot of time with your friends in the local community centre. Like most of your friends, you like to chew khat. You use up to about two bundles a day, on most days of the week. You share the cost with others. You are aware that its possession and use are not legal. You enjoy chewing it together with your friends and explain that it makes you feel happy. It makes you feel energetic and good about yourself.

Lately, you have been quite worried. You believe that your friends are spying on you and maybe passing on information about you to MI5. You think that people are talking about you in the street and you have heard people say things like: 'traitor' and 'kill him, kill him'. You are worried that you may be imprisoned and have become increasingly withdrawn.

10. Social phobia

You are a twenty-seven-year-old bachelor, who lives alone and works as a manager in an advertising agency. You have been off sick from work for the last week, and went to see your GP for a sick note. You told her that you wanted to be signed off for at least a few months as you are not ready to go back. Two months ago, you had attended one of the daily team meetings, and during a presentation, you had made a few mistakes. Some colleagues had laughed out aloud and you felt humiliated. You tried to ignore the episode, but over the next few weeks made excuses to avoid the meeting. Soon afterwards, you stopped going to the company meal area as you were worried that you might do something embarrassing.

At home, your mood has been low in the last week and, although you have found consolation in drinking alcohol, your intake has increased considerably. Whenever you have started getting ready to go to work, you have felt anxious, sweaty, and tremulous. Having been off work these last few days, you think you might not return at all.

You think that these fears are exaggerated, and that this is not like you at all, but want help for your problems.

11. Chronic fatigue syndrome

You are a thirty-five-year-old lady, who has been disabled by constant tiredness over the last year or so, which started soon after a bout of the 'flu. You used to work as a legal secretary, but had to give up work a few months after your tiredness began because you felt exhausted after each day's work, even though you were taking as much rest as possible. You started experiencing joint and muscle pains, and then recurrent headaches. You started thinking that your memory was failing you, and felt your concentration was also poor. In the last six months, you have spent most of your time at home, lying in bed, and have avoided any kind of activity. Your husband has become a full-time carer for you. Your GP, who has done many investigations, has now referred you to a psychiatrist, because he cannot find a medical cause for your symptoms.

12. Morbid jealousy

You are a forty-year-old married man, who lives with his wife and works at a grocery store. You have become convinced that your wife is being unfaithful to you, since finding a receipt for a large meal in her purse six months ago. Although she explained that this was for a working lunch meeting, you are sure she was out with her lover, whom you think might be her supervisor at work.

Over the last year, your relationship has deteriorated. Your excessive drinking has caused rows and in the last few months, you have not had a sexual relationship because you have found it difficult to sustain an erection. You are worried that your wife is seeking solace elsewhere.

Over the last two weeks, you have been following her to her workplace. You have been checking her purse, and looking through her clothes for any evidence of her infidelity.

As a last resort you thought that you should see your GP to ask if medication might help with your feelings of anger and resentment. He now wants you to see a psychiatrist.

13. Hypochondriasis

You are a forty-year-old man, with no previous history of mental illness. Two years ago you started to experience occasional headaches, which you initially thought were due to stress in your job as an accountant. Some months later you started thinking that there might be a more sinister cause, and in the last year you have become convinced that you have a brain tumour.

Since then, you have had numerous investigations, including a brain scan, via your GP and privately. You have even been seen by a neurologist, who did not find anything sinister. None of this has reassured you in any way. In the last week or so, you have noticed that your heart beats loudly whenever you do any physical work. You feel that this indicates that the tumour is worse and have been avoiding any form of exertion since.

You are spending more time looking up information on brain tumours on the internet. You have not felt particularly depressed, are not specifically anxious, and have not had any panic attacks or worries about any other illness. You have stopped talking with friends and family, as they are bored of you talking about your tumour incessantly. Your GP wants you to meet with a psychiatrist, but you are sceptical, as you are certain there is nothing 'wrong' with you from a mental health point of view.

14. Postnatal depression

You are a thirty-five-year-old postmistress, whose daughter was born four months ago. About five weeks after the birth, your mood dropped, and it has been low ever since. You have had difficulty sleeping and you feel tired all the time. You haven't been eating much and have lost three stone in weight. Everything has seemed an effort. In the last week, you have had fleeting thoughts of wanting to end your life, and you have actually thought of taking an overdose or hanging yourself. The only thing that has stopped you is the thought of your baby. Two nights ago, when the baby was crying, you came very close to throwing her out of the window of your two-storey flat. When you told your husband he took you to the GP immediately. You are now both here to see a psychiatrist. Your husband, who works as a teacher, has been off work for the last week as he is worried at your state. He is desperate for reassurance that you and the baby will be safe.

You will need to say at some stage that you would never harm your baby and that you would seek help from your husband or the GP if you had any thoughts of harming the baby again.

1.3

Instructions for examiners

1. Nightmares and night terrors

Introduces self.
Elicits relevant history, focussing on the pattern of sleep and sleep disruption.

Listening skills   A   B   C   D   E

Sensitivity   A   B   C   D   E

Question-framing   A   B   C   D   E

⌘ Explores role of stress in the presentation.

⌘ Explores relevant psychological factors.

Stress/psychological aspects   A   B   C   D   E

⌘ Considers and explores presence of epilepsy or brain tumour.

Medical aspects   A   B   C   D   E

Drugs and alcohol   A   B   C   D   E

⌘ Explains that sleep terrors and sleepwalking are closely related. Genetic, developmental, organic and psychological factors all play a role in their development, and the two conditions share the same clinical and patho-physiological characteristics.

Family history   A   B   C   D   E

Factual knowledge   A   B   C   D   E

Explains diagnosis   A   B   C   D   E

Ending   A   B   C   D   E

Global rating   A   B   C   D   E

Night terrors are different from nightmares. With night terrors, patients suddenly present in a state of severe anxiety, with a rapid heart rate and profuse sweating. If they wake they are usually confused, and are unable to recollect what caused them to wake up. Night terrors occur mainly in children but can present at any age. They tend to occur within the first hour of sleep. Nightmares, on the other hand, are not associated with intense autonomic disturbance. They usually occur in the second half of the sleep cycle, during REM sleep. Sufferers usually have a good memory for the nightmare.

2. Erectile dysfunction

Introduces self.
Explains reason for referral.

Introduction | A | | B | | C | | D | | E | |

⌘ Explores relevant aspects of history:

- onset and duration of problem
- aggravating and relieving factors
- fluctuations in the nature and severity of the problems
- overall quality of the sexual relationship
- smoking, alcohol and illicit drug use
- medical history, particularly diabetes mellitus, hypertension
- treatment for other physical problems, including medication
- history of back injury, operations, exposure to radiation.

⌘ Elicits past psychiatric history.

Empathy | A | | B | | C | | D | | E | |

Listening skills | A | | B | | C | | D | | E | |

Question-framing | A | | B | | C | | D | | E | |

⌘ Explores associated aspects of sexual history:

- extra marital relationships
- impact on the marital relationship and wife's viewpoint.

⌘ Elicits further details of presenting complaints:

- does he have erections — quality, duration, morning erections, frequency of sexual activity, time before ejaculation, ability to achieve orgasm, any concerns regarding the size of his penis or sexual performance, painful orgasm
- masturbatory activity — frequency, ability to have and sustain an erection.

Collateral history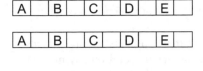

Screens for medical conditions

Differentiates organic and psychogenic erectile dysfunction

⌘ Explores emotional and other impact of symptoms:

- his and wife's perception of the problem, and their expectation for the future
- is the problem impacting on his daily occupational and social functioning?
- wife's current mental and physical health.

Emotional impact

Perception of problem

Elicits wife's history

Ending

Global rating

3. Forensic history

Introduces self.
Explains the purpose of the interview.
Is sensitive and empathic.
Listens to the patient.

Introduction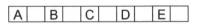

⌘ Elicits the relevant details of a forensic history:

- first caution, fine, charge, conviction, and imprisonment
- nature of charges and convictions
- duration of imprisonment
- probation sentences, related offences, related treatments
- did conditions include attendance at psychiatric services
- details of recorded offences
- details of unrecorded offences
- events preceding major offences.

⌘ Enquires about use of or possession of weapons.

⌘ Enquires about instances of fire setting or arson.

⌘ Enquires about violence to others:

- are there any outstanding charges?
- is he due in Court on any matter?
- how does he fund his habit? (an alternative to asking about current level of criminal activity)
- is he still involved in the supply of drugs to others?
- contact details of probation or any other service involved in his care.

Question-framing

A	B	C	D	E

Factual knowledge

A	B	C	D	E

⌘ What was the pattern in his offending behaviour? Is there an evidence of escalation in his offending behaviour? Has his behaviour deteriorated along with increase in his drug seeking behaviour?

⌘ What was the importance of the offences and the interplay between the prevailing mental state and offending behaviour? Was there any evidence of an illness at the time of the offences? Was it acquisitive in nature?

> It is important to cover a range of offences and ask about all interactions with police and other criminal justice system agencies. Specific enquiry should be made about non-convicted offences. Events surrounding offences should be investigated. Specific enquiry about the use of firearms and other weapons should be made. Candidate should focus on collecting information methodically.

Relevance of offences

A	B	C	D	E

Explores mental state at time of offences

A	B	C	D	E

⌘ What is his perception to the offences committed? How is he justifying his actions? Is he taking complete or partial responsibility for his actions? What does he feel about his victims? Is he showing any remorse? How is he planning to make changes to his life?

Explores attitude to offences

A	B	C	D	E

Ending

A	B	C	D	E

Global rating

A	B	C	D	E

4. Confusion and visual hallucinations

Introduces self.
Establishes rapport.

Explains the reason for the interview.
Is sensitive to the husband's distress.
Strikes a balance between open and closed questions.

Introduction |A| |B| |C| |D| |E| |

Communication |A| |B| |C| |D| |E| |

⌘ Inquires about circumstances that lead to the admission to hospital:

- similar episodes in the past
- duration
- progress.

⌘ Asks about level of consciousness:

- clouded
- fluctuating
- hyper-arousal.

Elicits relevant history |A| |B| |C| |D| |E| |

⌘ Assesses cognitive impairment:

- deficits in attention and concentration
- disorientation in time
- disorientation in place
- memory impairment
- slowness in thinking.

Brief cognitive assessment |A| |B| |C| |D| |E| |

⌘ Assesses psychotic symptoms:

- visual hallucinations
- other hallucinations
- delusional ideas
- elicits prevalent mood state.

Psychotic symptoms |A| |B| |C| |D| |E| |

⌘ History of physical illness:

- diabetes
- vascular illness
- CVAs or TIAs
- infections

- Parkinsonian symptoms.

Medical history |A| |B| |C| |D| |E| |

⌘ Current medication:

- analgesics
- steroids
- benzodiazepines
- beta-blockers
- digoxin
- antidepressants
- anticholinergic medication
- anti-parkinsonian medication.

Current medication |A| |B| |C| |D| |E| |

⌘ Elicits history of alcohol use:

- has she ever had any withdrawal symptoms?

Alcohol history |A| |B| |C| |D| |E| |

⌘ Summarizes and explains the need for further assessment, care and treatment.

⌘ Considers delirium, Lewy body or other forms of dementia in the discussion with the husband.

⌘ Explains the need for physical examination and blood and urine tests.

Summarization |A| |B| |C| |D| |E| |

Ending |A| |B| |C| |D| |E| |

Global rating |A| |B| |C| |D| |E| |

5. Depression with psychotic symptoms

Introduces self.
Establishes rapport.
Shows empathy.
Is sensitive to the patients distress.
Establishes a balance between open and closed questions.

Communication |A| |B| |C| |D| |E| |

Question-framing   A | B | C | D | E |

⌘ Enquires about mood:

- lack of energy
- lack of interest/anhedonia
- self-care.

Mood symptoms   A | B | C | D | E |

⌘ Asks about biological symptoms:

- appetite
- weight-loss
- constipation
- early morning waking
- worsening of mood in the morning.

Biological symptoms   A | B | C | D | E |

⌘ Enquires about nihilistic delusions, guilt, paranoid ideas:

> *Is there anything you are worried about? Do you have any worries/concerns?*
> *What about your health?*
> *Are you worried about your health in any way?*
> *Do you have any concerns that your body is not functioning in the way that it should?*
> *Do you have any worries about your financial situation? Are you able to pay your bills? Do you have any debts?*
> *Do you blame yourself for anything you have done? Do you think that you have done anything wrong? Do you feel guilty about it?*
> *What do other people say about you? Does anyone criticise you in any way?*

Nihilistic delusions   A | B | C | D | E |

Guilt   A | B | C | D | E |

⌘ Enquires about hallucinations:

> *Have you seen or heard anything that you could not explain?*
> *Has there been anything else that you have experienced that you could not explain, such as tasting or smelling anything unusual?*

Hallucinations   A | B | C | D | E |

⌘ Performs a risk assessment:

> *Do you ever feel that these worries are more than you can bear? Have you ever felt that it is too much for you?*
> *Do you feel your life is still worth living? Have you ever felt that it would be better if you were not around?*
> *Have you ever felt like ending it all/your life?*
> *Have you made any plans? Have you talked to anyone else about this?*

Risk assessment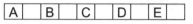

⌘ Summarizes and concludes the interview.

⌘ Explains need for further exploration.

⌘ Suggests treatment options.

Ending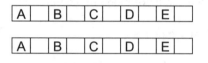

Global rating

6. Excessive day-time sleepiness

Introduces self.
Explains reason for the interview.
Establishes rapport.
Uses open and closed questions.

Introduction

Communication

Question-framing

⌘ Elicits a history of sleep problems:

- duration of sleep
- initial insomnia
- time of waking
- sleep arrangements
- quality of sleep
- dreaming
- bed-time routine
- use of coffee, tea and cola
- alcohol use.

Sleep history | A | | B | | C | | D | | E | |

⌘ Checks for factors related to obstructive sleep apnoea:

- heavy snoring
- irregular breathing in sleep
- overweight
- alcohol use
- nasal septum deviation
- nasal allergies/adenoids.

⌘ Elicits symptoms of narcolepsy:

- episodes of sudden daytime sleepiness
- presence of sudden muscle weakness (cataplexy) triggered by emotions
- visual or auditory hallucinations while falling asleep (hypnagogic hallucinations)
- episodes of inability to move while falling asleep or waking (sleep-paralysis).

Elicits symptoms | A | | B | | C | | D | | E | |

Considers different diagnoses | A | | B | | C | | D | | E | |

⌘ Points out risk of falling asleep while

- driving
- operating machinery

Risk assessment | A | | B | | C | | D | | E | |

⌘ Gives specific advice:

- try to lose weight
- avoid alcohol before going to sleep
- consider referral to a chest-physician or ENT surgeon
- use of a constant positive airway pressure (CPAP) machine at night, 'which blows a gentle stream of air through the nose, which prevents the throat from narrowing whilst breathing in.'

General sleep hygiene | A | | B | | C | | D | | E | |

Considers further management | A | | B | | C | | D | | E | |

Ending | A | | B | | C | | D | | E | |

Global rating | A | | B | | C | | D | | E | |

7. Chronic pain

Introduces self.
Establishes rapport.
Uses open and closed questions.

Communication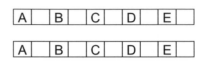

Question-framing

⌘ Elicits a history of the abdominal pain:

> *Can you tell me something more about your problem?*
> *When did it start/how long has it been going on for? How has it developed over time?*
> *Can you describe the pain? Is it a dull, sharp, stabbing, or cramping type of pain?*
> *Where is it located?*
> *Do you have any other problems with your physical health?*
> *What about your bowel-movements?*
> *Do you have an explanation for the pain?*
> *Is there anything else that could have played a role?*

History of the pain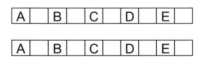

Associated symptoms

⌘ Assesses associated factors:

> *Is there anything that makes it worse? How does your mood/stress affect the pain?*
> *What sorts of investigations have you had? What were the results? Have the negative results reassured you? Why not?*
> *Have you had any treatment? Was it helpful? Is there anything else that has been helpful?*
> *Have you been told what is wrong with you? What is your understanding of what is wrong?*
> *How has it affected your mood?*
> *Has it affected the relationship with your wife and children?*
> *Do you have any specific worries with regard to the pain? Are you worried that there may be something seriously wrong with you?*

Psycho-social factors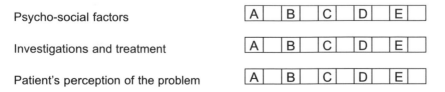

Investigations and treatment

Patient's perception of the problem

⌘ Acknowledges the reality of the pain.

⌘ Picks up on cues that emotional or psycho-social factors may play a role.

⌘ Explains the influence of depression, anxiety and stress on the symptoms.

Explains role of other factors | A | B | C | D | E |

⌘ Gives specific advice on:

- smaller portions of food
- fibre-rich food
- stress-management
- relaxation
- cognitive behavioural therapy (CBT)
- yoga
- counselling
- antidepressants, such as low dose amitriptyline.

General advice | A | B | C | D | E |

Explores treatment options | A | B | C | D | E |

Ending | A | B | C | D | E |

Global rating | A | B | C | D | E |

8. History of an epileptic seizure

Introduces self.
Takes a clear and relevant history.

Communication | A | B | C | D | E |

Question-framing | A | B | C | D | E |

⌘ Assesses post-ictal confusion:

- level of consciousness
- disorientation
- amnesia for the event.

Assessment of confusion | A | B | C | D | E |

⌘ Post-ictal signs, include:

- incontinence
- tongue bite
- head-injury
- other injuries
- focal neurological deficits.

Post-ictal signs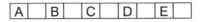

⌘ Elicits:

- past history of epilepsy or fits
- previous history of epilepsy, particularly absences and tonic-clonic seizures
- last seizure? Where? Was it observed? What was done at the time?
- investigations done
- presence of prodromal period
- presence of an aura.

History

⌘ Use of substances:

- alcohol (rum-fits)
- alcohol withdrawal
- illicit drug use, including cocaine and amphetamines.

Alcohol and drug history

⌘ Use of drugs that lower the seizure threshold:

- antipsychotics, eg. chlorpromazine
- tricyclic antidepressants, eg. amitriptyline
- other antidepressants

⌘ Stopping drugs that increase the seizure threshold:

- benzodiazepines
- anti-epileptic drugs, eg. carbamazepine, sodium valproate

Role of medication

⌘ Exposure to seizure-inducing stimuli:

- lack of sleep
- flashes of light on TV or computer game
- hyperventilation.

⌘ Considers other causes:

- head injury
- hypertension
- vascular causes
- metabolic causes
- infections.

Other causes   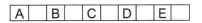

⌘ Summarizes and explains the need for further investigations.

Summary and ending | A | B | C | D | E |

Global rating | A | B | C | D | E |

9. Substance-induced psychosis

Introduces self.
Establishes rapport.
Is non-judgmental.
Shows sensitivity to patient's background and situation.
Establishes a balance between open and closed questions.

Communication | A | B | C | D | E |

Question-framing | A | B | C | D | E |

⌘ Obtains information regarding patient's background.

⌘ Takes a relevant history of the current symptoms:

- presence of delusions
- content
- presence of hallucinations
- type of hallucinations
- content
- duration of symptoms
- past history
- precipitating factors.

History   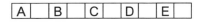

⌘ Asks about substance misuse:

- alcohol

- cannabis
- amphetamines
- cocaine
- khat.

General substance use   A | B | C | D | E |

⌘ Elicits history of khat use (Cox and Rampes, 2003):

- duration of use
- frequency
- amount consumed
- cultural context
- supply
- funding
- features of dependence
- effects.

History of khat use   A | B | C | D | E |

⌘ Psychological effects:

- euphoria
- excitement
- increased levels of energy
- increased ability to concentrate
- improved self-esteem
- delayed effects
- insomnia
- lack of concentration
- low mood.

Psychological effects of use   A | B | C | D | E |

⌘ Physical effects of khat:

- dry mouth
- polydipsia
- anorexia
- weight-loss
- tachycardia
- hypertension.

Physical effects of use   A | B | C | D | E |

⌘ Suggests possible connection between psychosis and khat use.

⌘ Explores patient's perception of the problem.

⌘ Examines insight and motivation to change.

Patient's perception of problem |A| |B| |C| |D| |E| |

Assessment of motivation to change |A| |B| |C| |D| |E| |

Ending |A| |B| |C| |D| |E| |

Global rating |A| |B| |C| |D| |E| |

10. Social phobia

Introduces him/herself.
Shows empathy and respect.
Asks open and closed questions.

Introduction |A| |B| |C| |D| |E| |

Question-framing |A| |B| |C| |D| |E| |

Verbal facilitation |A| |B| |C| |D| |E| |

⌘ Explores symptom history, precipitating factors and associated problems:

> *Can you tell me how this problem started? What happened after that?*
> *What happens when you start getting ready to go back to work?*

Assesses symptom onset
and progression |A| |B| |C| |D| |E| |

⌘ Elicits diagnostic criteria for social phobia:

> *What happens when you want to go for a meeting? Have you in any way*
> *tried to avoid the situations that cause you anxiety?*
> *Did your anxiety ever get out of control? What sort of things happened to*
> *you then?*
> *Are you anxious only when you need to go for a meeting or a meal with*
> *others?*
> *Do you feel similarly anxious in any other situation?*
> *How have you tried to deal with this anxiety? How has it affected your life?*

Checks social phobia symptoms |A| |B| |C| |D| |E| |

⌘ Asks about associated symptoms, such as:

- shaking, nausea, blushing, wanting to use the toilet
- anxiety in other situations, such as writing in public, using public toilets, or other social situations, such as parties or conferences.

Associated symptoms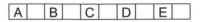

⌘ Explores comorbid conditions:

- depression, including suicidal thoughts or plans
- alcohol and drug abuse, (and excessive caffeine intake) and if time permits, assess if dependence is an issue
- obsessive compulsive disorder.

⌘ Explores family history of similar or related mental illnesses.

⌘ Ask about phobias, depression, and alcohol and drug abuse in the family.

Explores comorbidity and family history [A] [B] [C] [D] [E]

⌘ Discusses likely diagnosis and common investigations:

What you have described are symptoms of an illness that is called social phobia. It is an illness, because unlike 'normal' social anxiety, your symptoms are interfering with your occupational and even social functioning. Some of your relatives might be affected by similar symptoms. The anxiety leads to attempts to avoid the feared situation, in your case the regular meetings, and can later extend to other situations. It is common for sufferers to use alcohol and even illicit drugs as a way of coping with the anxiety. We will, of course, need to perform some routine tests, including blood tests and an ECG, a tracing of the electrical activity of your heart, to make sure we rule out any physical illness that might present with the same symptoms. I will also give you a leaflet about anxiety; what you may experience, and how you can learn to deal with it.

⌘ Discusses the various non-pharmacological treatments that are available:

- anxiety management techniques
- breathing control and relaxation exercises
- re-learning and practice of conversational and social skills
- graded exposure, using a hierarchy of feared situations
- cognitive behavioural therapy.

⌘ Discusses the various pharmacological treatments that are available:

- selective serotonin reuptake inhibitors (SSRIs) — paroxetine, fluoxetine, sertraline, or citalopram

- beta-blockers to augment antidepressant therapy for performance anxiety and non-generalised social phobia.

Discusses diagnosis and investigations | A | B | C | D | E |

Discusses treatment options | A | B | C | D | E |

Addresses patient's concerns | A | B | C | D | E |

Global rating | A | B | C | D | E |

11. Chronic fatigue syndrome (CFS)

Introduces self, explains reason for seeing a psychiatrist:

Hello Mrs Blaine. Your GP sent you here to see if we can help with the constant tiredness or fatigue you have been experiencing. I know you have had numerous investigations, and I will have a look at the results shortly, but I'd like to start by asking you how and when all of this began.

Introduction | A | B | C | D | E |

Sensitivity | A | B | C | D | E |

The main point is to elicit whether she has symptoms that would fulfil the current case criteria for chronic fatigue syndrome. These include:

1. Chronic, medically unexplained fatigue of at least six month's duration, which has not been a lifelong problem, is not due to continuing exertion, is not wholly relieved by rest, and is associated with a reduction in previous level of activities.
2. Four or more of the following: subjective memory impairment; sore throat; tender lymph nodes; muscle pain; joint pain; headache; unrefreshing sleep; post-exertional malaise lasting more than twenty-four hours.
3. And, excluding active or unresolved physical disease: psychotic depression; depression with somatic syndrome; and depressive episode within a bipolar illness; other psychotic disorder; dementia; anorexia of bulimia nervosa; alcohol or substance misuse; severe obesity (these would probably best be screened using just single questions, or observation, or common sense in the case of dementia, because you don't have the time to examine these in depth during the OSCE).

Ideally, it would be useful to explore the main symptom, namely the fatigue, particularly looking for its onset, duration and progress. Unfortunately, the criteria do not exclude uncomplicated depression, so you should try to cover at least the three main diagnostic criteria for depression (persistent low mood, low energy levels, and anhedonia), as well as some biological symptoms.

⌘ Clarifies the presenting complaints and excludes important differential diagnoses.

Assesses fatigue onset, duration and progression
     A☐ B☐ C☐ D☐ E☐

Elicits associated symptoms
     A☐ B☐ C☐ D☐ E☐

Excludes other illnesses
     A☐ B☐ C☐ D☐ E☐

⌘ Explains to the patient about the provisional diagnosis that has been made.

⌘ Discusses the initial steps in management, starting with investigations.

> At this stage it is essential to use simple language. Chronic fatigue syndrome (CFS) can be described as a, 'collection of symptoms characterized by disabling fatigue, made worse by exertion. It is also known as 'ME' (myalgic encephalitis) or 'post-viral fatigue'. There are many possible causal factors, such as viral illnesses and stress, but no one single cause has yet been identified. Based on what is already known of the associated problems such as loss of physical fitness, there are many suggested treatments, including talking therapies such as cognitive behavioural therapy, and programmes of graded exercise to try to get patients gradually to return to avoided activities.
> The key point is to reassure the patient that these symptoms are now recognized as a clinical problem that has both medical and psychological aspects. Remember that patients with CFS tend to believe that it is a purely medical illness, and you can say that whilst you acknowledge her beliefs without necessarily agreeing with them, you will need to work together in a collaborative approach to managing the problem.

It would be useful to state that you would need to have a look at the investigations the patient has already had (but bearing in mind that you would only investigate further if new clinical signs appear). Mention that you would focus on identifying any psychiatric illness, particularly depression, and anxiety disorder, and would assess the suicide risk. Also, mention that you would examine in more detail her illness beliefs, coping behaviour, occupational and interpersonal problems.

Explanation of diagnosis
     A☐ B☐ C☐ D☐ E☐

Initial investigations
     A☐ B☐ C☐ D☐ E☐

⌘ Discusses further management, and addresses concerns.

Say that you accept her symptoms as genuine, and that you will provide further education on the syndrome. Mention that you will treat any identifiable depression or anxiety. Your focus in treatment will be to assist her to return to normal functioning by looking at her avoidance of activity, and using structured, incremental exercises to facilitate physical activity. Ask her if she has any questions or concerns, and try to address them (for further information see Fukuda *et al*, 1994).

Further management   [A] [B] [C] [D] [E]

Addresses concerns   [A] [B] [C] [D] [E]

Ending   [A] [B] [C] [D] [E]

Global rating   [A] [B] [C] [D] [E]

12. Morbid jealousy

Introduces self.
Asks open and closed questions.
This is a difficult scenario, and must be approached with care. From the history you have been given, you might already be thinking of delusional jealousy. The key point is that the only informant you have is the patient in front of you. You will therefore have to facilitate his talking to you, using open questions and a non-judgmental approach:

> *I wonder if we could start by looking at what has happened for you to need medication. Would you tell me how all of this began?*

Introduction   [A] [B] [C] [D] [E]

Question-framing   [A] [B] [C] [D] [E]

Verbal facilitation   [A] [B] [C] [D] [E]

⌘ Explores symptom history, precipitating factors and associated problems:

> *Can you tell me more about your suspicions? What evidence have you had of her unfaithfulness?*
> *What sort of things have you been doing to check up on your wife?*
> *Have you been following her?*
> *How has your mood been recently? And what about your sleep and appetite?*

Elicits presenting complaints   [A] [B] [C] [D] [E]

⌘ Explores the actual quality of his beliefs:

> *How convinced are you that she is having an affair?*
> *What if I said that you are only misinterpreting what has been happening, and that it all sounds innocent to me?*

How much of your time has been spent looking for evidence?

⌘ Apart from what is happening now, is he usually an over possessive partner? Have there been previous episodes of jealousy, and how has he reacted?

Elicits nature and severity of beliefs |A| |B| |C| |D| |E|

⌘ Elicits any underlying mental illness or other associated problems.

You will need to need quickly to screen for schizophrenia (for example, by asking for paranoid beliefs, and abnormal perceptions), mood disorders (either depression or mania), obsessive compulsive disorder (OCD), personality disorder (especially paranoid, antisocial, borderline, histrionic and narcissistic types), and alcohol and substance misuse (especially looking for dependence criteria in this case). The more difficult aspects to consider are actual marital or sexual problems in the relationship. You should ask about them, and elaborate on the sexual dysfunction issues, but remember that to get an accurate picture, a collateral history is vital.
You might not get any indication of other underlying mental illness, and will then have to consider that the patient has a delusional disorder of the jealousy subtype.

Elicits underlying mental illness |A| |B| |C| |D| |E|

⌘ Assesses the level of risk posed to partner:

- how have feelings towards his wife been affected by his behaviour? Is he angry or resentful?
- how often does he interrogate her? Has any confrontation occurred?
- if not, has he thought of confronting her? How has she responded to his accusations?
- has there been any violence so far? Has he thought about what he might do if his fears are proved correct?
- has there been any previous violence in their relationship?

Assesses risk   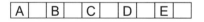 |A| |B| |C| |D| |E|

⌘ Discusses further management.

The first step would be to get a collateral history. However this is not possible in the OSCE setting, so you would probably need to discuss the further management of the case as if you have confirmed your diagnosis. Tactfully suggest that, although you can understand what he has said, you are worried that his jealous thinking and behaviour are unreasonable in their intensity, and that they are impeding his normal everyday life. Avoid confrontation, but suggest that there are many ways in which he might get help with the problem. You could mention the option of medication, and talking therapy such as cognitive behavioural therapy. Ask if he has any questions or concerns.

Discusses initial findings and possible therapy

A	B	C	D	E

Addresses patient's concerns

A	B	C	D	E

Global rating

A	B	C	D	E

13. Hypochondriasis

Introduces self, and explains reason for meeting with a psychiatrist.

> *Hello, Mr Brown. Your GP has asked me to meet with you to talk about your headaches and the concerns you have that you may have a brain tumour. Could we perhaps start by talking about how your headaches have been lately?*

The key point to remember is that he is probably tired of trying to convince his doctors/family/friends, is wary of talking to a psychiatrist, and only wants to focus on the physical aspects of his presentation. Your strategy is to start by focusing on what he is interested in talking about. Once you have established some rapport, you can ask more focused questions.

Introduction

A	B	C	D	E

Establishes rapport

A	B	C	D	E

Tactful questioning

A	B	C	D	E

⌘ Explores the preoccupation with fear of having a brain tumour (symptom onset, duration and progress):

- how and when did he start having thoughts along these lines?
- is the patient anxious that he may have a tumour or is he convinced that he has one? What leads him to feel that he has a tumour? Are there any specific symptoms that convince him? How does he know these are due to the 'tumour?' Could he summarise the results of tests that he has had so far?

⌘ Explores the fixity of the illness belief (severity and frequency of current symptoms):

- how certain is he that he has a tumour? Has he heard or read about anything that might explain how he came to believe this about himself?
- is there any other explanation for each symptom or the symptoms in combination? What about the reassurances given by his doctors?

⌘ Assesses impact on activities of daily living and quality of life:

- what sorts of thoughts does he have every day? How much of his daily life is affected by his preoccupation with illness? In what ways does he seek reassurance? How has he been getting on with his doctor? What about his relationships with family and friends?

⌘ Explores specific issues within the history:

- has there been any history of traumatic events or early childhood illness? Was he a sick child, or was he often absent from school on grounds of illness?
- has he experienced any stressful life events lately? Has anyone in the family or someone he knows been ill or died in similar circumstances?

The point to remember is that in hypochondriasis, the beliefs about a serious disease are over-valued beliefs, and make some sense in terms of the patient's experience.

Presenting complaints   A B C D E

Over-valued beliefs   A B C D E

Impact of symptoms   A B C D E

Relevant personal history   A B C D E

⌘ Explores associated symptoms:

- does he have specific fears about dying or death? How concerned is he with his overall health?
- does he repeatedly examine or monitor himself in any way? Has he stopped doing anything because of his beliefs? Does he avoid doing anything because of his worries?

⌘ Explores comorbid conditions and addresses differential diagnoses.

This is difficult because of the overlap of symptoms. The main comorbid conditions, namely depression and anxiety disorders, are also the main differentials. If there is time, try to establish whether the hypochondriasis is primary or secondary, ie, what came first? If there isn't the time, at least ask brief screening questions for depression, anxiety, and psychotic disorders.

Associated symptoms   A B C D E

Comorbid conditions   A B C D E

Differential diagnoses   A B C D E

⌘ Summarizes the findings and explain the diagnosis.

Remember, you are still trying to establish a therapeutic relationship (albeit in the setting of an exam). You might start by summarising the presenting complaints, and any other comorbidity you may have elicited. Then state that you will need to work together to tackle the problem. Explain that the main options that have helped people 'with similar problems' are talking therapies or medication. Ask whether he would like to know more. If so, explain that the talking therapies such as cognitive behavioural therapy look at identifying misinterpretation of symptoms and thought processes about illness, and try to modify wrongful assumptions and identify more realistic interpretations. They may also involve graded exposure to feared situations, and prevention of reassurance-seeking behaviour. On the other hand, medications such as antidepressants have also been shown to be effective. The main focus will be to work together; regular reviews (not related to the onset/worsening of symptoms) might be a useful start. Also, you can say that you do not feel that further investigations are indicated at this stage and that you will be working closely with his GP and neurologist to find what works. Ask if he has any questions or concerns and try to answer them briefly.

Summarisation | A | B | C | D | E |

Addresses patient's concerns | A | B | C | D | E |

Ending | A | B | C | D | E |

Global rating | A | B | C | D | E |

14. Postnatal depression

Introduces self, explains reason for seeing a psychiatrist:

> *Hello Mr and Mrs Daniels. My name is Dr Michael. I am one of the psychiatrists here. Your GP has asked me to see you, to see if there is anything we could help you with. Could I start by asking whether you are happy for me to conduct this interview with your husband present?*

Introductions | A | B | C | D | E |

Confidential issues | A | B | C | D | E |

⌘ Clarifies the presenting complaints (see also, *Objective Structed Clinical Examination for Psychiatric Trainees*, volume I: question 8):

- prevailing mood, energy levels, and interests.

⌘ Asks about changes in biological functions:

How have you been feeling in yourself lately?
What about your energy levels?
Do you feel unusually tired during the day?
Have you been enjoying activities as much recently?
What has your sleep been like? Do you have difficulty getting off to sleep?
Do you sleep the whole way through the night?
Are you able to concentrate on tasks?
Have you had any difficulty reading or watching television?
What about your interest in sex? Has that been affected in any way?

⌘ Has she ever suffered from depression or other mental illness before? Has she needed treatment or hospitalisation?

History of mood change   A ☐ B ☐ C ☐ D ☐ E ☐

Biological symptoms   A ☐ B ☐ C ☐ D ☐ E ☐

Past psychiatric history   A ☐ B ☐ C ☐ D ☐ E ☐

⌘ Explores temporal relationship of symptoms with childbirth.

⌘ Explore the onset, duration and progression of depressed mood:

- how soon after the birth did she first notice that her mood was low? Did her husband notice it as well? Did she mention it to the health visitor or GP?
- has she been overly concerned with the baby's health?
- has she been worried about an inability to cope? Has she had enough support during the postpartum period? Have there been any other social stresses in the life? How supportive has her husband been? How are they getting on now?

> The key point is to distinguish the later onset of postnatal depression (five to six weeks postnatal) from the earlier onset of the 'postnatal / baby blues' (third to fifth day). The 'blues' is considered to be a brief time-limited period of psychological disturbance, which normally resolves by itself and needs only reassurance and support. On the other hand, postnatal depression, though phenomenologically not different from clinical depression, is thought to be associated with recent stressful life events, younger age, poor marital relationship, absent social support, and a past history of depression. Postpartum psychosis is effectively ruled out from the history given, but it may be worth enquiring about perplexity, restlessness, anxiety and insomnia, and also affective fluctuation with delusions and hallucinations that may have arisen abruptly within the first two weeks of childbirth.

Temporal relationship with childbirth   A ☐ B ☐ C ☐ D ☐ E ☐

Stresses and supports   A ☐ B ☐ C ☐ D ☐ E ☐

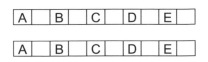

Diagnostic criteria | A | | B | | C | | D | | E | |

❋ Examines risks to mother and child.

Although you are going to be concerned about the risk to mother and child, it would seem more appropriate to explore these issues once you have established some rapport with the more general questions, as above.

> *I understand that you have had thoughts of wanting to end your life. Could you tell me more about these thoughts? Have you made any plans? How close have you come to carrying out your plans?*
> *I understand you have also said that you had thoughts of throwing the baby out of the window. I know how distressing these thoughts can be, but can you tell me more about them? How close have you come to doing so? What stopped you? If it happens again, what do you think you will do? Have you thought of harming the baby in any other way?*

❋ Asks husband his impression of the risks to mother and child.

Explores main risks | A | | B | | C | | D | | E | |

❋ Summarizes the findings and diagnosis .

The key point is to mention that she appears to have symptoms of postnatal depression, and that this is more than what would be expected for a new mother. Explain that this is more than just a simple low mood and is clearly affecting her capacity to enjoy life, and also the routine functions of life like sleeping and eating. Mention her thoughts of ending her life or that of her child.

❋ Explains the main options at this stage.

Firstly you can say that, in view of the risks expressed regarding her child, you will have to speak to your social work colleagues now for their advice. You should say that one option is a period of inpatient assessment and treatment. State that if she agrees, you would then have to discuss it with your consultant. She might need a placement at the local mother and baby unit. Secondly, if she refuses admission, say that you would have to consider follow up by a community psychiatric nurse (CPN) at the outpatient clinic, along with any monitoring your social work colleagues might consider necessary. Say that you will give her a leaflet explaining postnatal depression and the help that is available. Ask her if she has any questions.

Summarizations | A | | B | | C | | D | | E | |

Initial managements | A | | B | | C | | D | | E | |

Addresses patient's concerns | A | | B | | C | | D | | E | |

Ending | A | | B | | C | | D | | E | |

Global rating | A | | B | | C | | D | | E | |

References

Cox G, Rampes H (2003) Adverse effects of khat: a review. *Adv Psychiatric Treatment* **9**: 546–63

Fukuda K, Strauss SE, Hickie IB, Sharpe M, Dobbins JG, Komaroff AL (1994) Chronic fatigue syndrome: a comprehensive approach to its definition and management. *Ann Int Med* **121**: 953–9

Section two:
Examination and procedural skills

2.1

Instructions for candidates

---

15. Assessment for inpatient detention

You are called to assess an inpatient at your local psychiatric unit on a Saturday. This twenty-two-year-old man has been in hospital for four days and has been detained under the Nurses' Emergency detention powers (Section 5(4) in England and Wales) for the past hour as he was found trying to leave the ward. The working diagnosis is of psychotic depression and he has refused to take his prescribed medication over the past twenty-four hours. He had suicidal thoughts at the time of admission.

Assess the patient for further detention and advise staff on further management.

16. Assessment of motivation to change

You are in the psychiatric outpatient clinic. Your next patient wants you to consider him for a trial of acamprosate.

Assess his motivation to change.

17. Risk assessment in dementia

This forty-eight-year-old woman works as a full-time solicitor, and has asked to speak to you. She would like to discuss the concerns she has about her mother who has dementia. Her parents used to manage fairly well together but her father recently died of an aortic aneurysm. Her mother has been living on her own since and is not coping well.

Assess the relevant risks from this informant and address her concerns.

18. Bulimia nervosa

You are asked to see a twenty-year-old lady, who works as a receptionist, in your outpatient clinic. She has been referred by her GP who is concerned that she has asked for help to lose weight, after admitting that she has been inducing vomiting in an effort to keep her weight down. Her weight is within the normal range, but she seems preoccupied with it, and has even asked for a prescription of laxatives.

Assess this patient for symptoms and signs of bulimia nervosa.

19. Management of acute dystonia

You are asked to see a patient urgently on your ward. A staff nurse reported that this twenty-one-year-old man had suddenly become breathless, and complained his tongue was swollen.

Assess the situation and instruct nursing staff accordingly.

20. Rapid tranquillisation

You are called to see a patient in the intensive care unit of your hospital. He has been physically restrained and is being nursed in a side-room according to local seclusion policy. Earlier, nursing staff had been concerned about his verbal aggression and had had to move him away from another patient. They had tried verbal reassurance and de-escalation techniques, without much success.

Assess him and manage the situation appropriately.

21. Drug interactions

A fifty-year-old lady, currently an inpatient on this ward, visited the dentist and had her tooth extracted yesterday. The duty psychiatrist commenced her on ibuprofen for pain relief. Nursing staff have asked you to see her as she has appeared drowsy all morning, and is complaining of swelling around her eyes and ankles and stiffness in her arms and legs. Her blood pressure an hour ago was 80/50mm Hg. However, she was given her morning medication.

Examine her prescription card carefully and discuss any potential concerns.

22. An agitated patient

You are asked to see this thirty-two-year-old single man, who suffers from schizophrenia. He was taken to the local Accident & Emergency Department (A&E) by the police after he assaulted a stranger in the street. The staff members in A&E feel that he is paranoid and are finding it difficult to manage him.

Assess the patient and try to contain the situation.

23. Lower limb function

Test tone, power, sensation (apart from pain and temperature) and coordination in this patient's legs.

24. Head injury

You are asked to urgently see this sixty-five-year-old female patient on the psychiatric ward. She was admitted for depressive symptoms and was started on an antidepressant some days ago.

This morning, she fell over when she got out of bed and hit her head on a radiator. When the nursing staff checked on her, they found her unconscious, but breathing normally.

Assess the severity of her head injury.

25. Apraxia, agnosia and Gerstmann's syndrome

This sixty-five-year-old man has had several small cerebrovascular accidents in the last year. He has difficulties with practical skills, such as eating, dressing and self-care.

Assess him for apraxia, agnosia and Gerstmann's syndrome.

26. Korsakov's syndrome

You are asked to see this fifty-year-old man, who has a long history of heavy alcohol consumption.

Six months ago he was admitted with acute confusion, ataxia and nystagmus. He was treated with multi vitamins but, in spite of this, he continues to have a degree of amnesia.

Assess this patient for symptoms of Korsakov's syndrome.

27. Cardiopulmonary resuscitation

This patient (represented by the manikin) has collapsed on the ward. Nursing Staff have crash bleeped you from the next ward.

Commence cardio-pulmonary resuscitation.

28. Electroconvulsive therapy (ECT) procedure

You are asked by your consultant to administer ECT to this patient. Your patient (represented by this manikin) has been prepared for the procedure by the staff nurse on the ward.

Administer one dose of ECT to this patient.

29. Language and non-dominant hemisphere functions

You have been asked to see a forty-seven-year-old man, with a year's history of progressive word-finding difficulties and impaired verbal and written comprehension. It is suspected that he suffers from temporal lobe dysfunction as a result of Pick's disease.

Assess his language and non-dominant hemisphere functions.

2.2

Instructions for actors

---

15. Assessment for inpatient detention

You are a twenty-two-year-old single salesman, and live with your parents. You have been feeling depressed for the past few months, and your mood became so low that you could not continue at work. You lost all interest in life. You have been feeling responsible for the wars in Iraq, Somalia and Bosnia. You feel as if you are a burden on the State and have not claimed social security benefits. You have lost about 7 kg in weight over the past few months. You have been unable to sleep, and have been isolating yourself at home.

A month ago, your parents took you to the GP who prescribed an antidepressant. You didn't take it, because you felt you were wasting the resources of the Health Service. In the last week, your mood has plummeted. When you talked about having suicidal thoughts such as jumping in front of a train, your parents became very worried and brought you to hospital for assessment.

Since being admitted, there has been no change in your mood. You feel guilty for taking a bed that could be used for someone else. You feel you're wasting everyone's time, and that you would be better off dead. Earlier today, you decided to go home and take an overdose of paracetamol tablets. You were stopped by the nursing staff when you tried to leave hospital, because they said that they were concerned about you. You are surprised at all the fuss being made .

16. Assessment of motivation to change

You are twenty-four-year-old married man who lives with his supportive, teetotal wife and two children. Your alcohol use began in your early teens, and has gradually increased, until you were spending around £120 per week, mostly on spirits. Your wife left you briefly due to frequent rows and you thought that this was the final chance you had to give up alcohol for good. You had an inpatient detoxification from alcohol at your local psychiatric hospital six weeks ago, and you have remained abstinent since. You have had three previous inpatient admissions for the same treatment; though this is the longest you have been 'dry'. You have been attending local Alcoholics Anonymous meetings, and have also seen your keyworker at the community alcohol service for direct counselling sessions. With her help, you have even interviewed for a job at a local supermarket. You did inform your prospective employers of your alcohol problem.

You have heard of a new wonder drug called acamprosate, which promises to reduce the powerful cravings you still get for alcohol, and hope that taking it will help you save your marriage and your future.

17. Risk assessment in dementia

You are a forty-eight-year-old lady, with a busy, full-time job as a solicitor. You are divorced and have two sons, who are at university. Your mother is seventy-five years old and has been suffering from dementia for the last three years. Your father used to take care of her, but died unexpectedly two months ago of an aortic aneurysm. Your mother has been living alone since and you are very concerned about her situation. You live in the same town and try to visit every day, but find it hard to combine this with your busy job.

You have been bringing her pre-prepared meals, which she can heat up in the micro-wave oven, but you have found food untouched in the fridge on several occasions. Your mother used to take pride in her appearance, but since your father's death she has been neglecting her self, and sometimes, her clothes have smelt of urine. You offered to help her with the laundry but she refused, saying she was able to take care of herself. Once, when you tried to make her remove some of her dirty clothes, she scratched you. She is physically well and has not had any falls. You have sometimes found her looking around the house for your father, but she has not wandered outside as yet. She has phoned you at night on some occasions to ask where your father is.

You wonder whether she might be better of in a residential home.

18. Bulimia nervosa

You are a twenty-year-old female hotel receptionist. Your GP has asked you to see a psychiatrist after you asked for laxatives to help you lose weight. Although your weight is within the normal range for your height, you have decided that you would like to weigh a lot less. Over the last year, you feel you have lost control of your eating, and have been eating in massive binges, once in two or three days. After each such meal, you have made yourself sick. You are scared of becoming 'fat'. You have read about bulimia in the newspapers, and want to know if this is what you suffer from.

19. Management of acute dystonia

You are a twenty-one-year-old man, and are currently an inpatient in the local psychiatric unit. This is your first admission to a psychiatric hospital. You were admitted after responding to frightening voices in your head by jumping in front of a moving car. After the doctor saw you on the ward, you were written up for a drug called haloperidol. You had your first dose of this medication about six hours ago and the second dose about an hour ago.

In the last half an hour, you have suddenly developed muscular spasms in your neck and your head is now fully tilted to one side. Your eyes are also turned up to the same side and you cannot bring them back to normal. You have just told the nurse that your tongue feels swollen, and she has summoned a doctor urgently. You are extremely frightened.

If there is an actor representing a nurse, this person is also asked to familiarise themselves with the above history. When asked, repeat relevant parts of the history and follow any instructions given.

20. Rapid tranquillisation

You are a twenty-four-year-old single man, currently an inpatient on this psychiatric unit. You are lying face down on the floor of the room, being restrained by four nurses. You are frightened and angry.

21. Drug interactions

The candidate will address the examiner directly. A copy of the *British National Formulary* (*BNF*) is available for the candidate.

Medication	Dose	Frequency	Route
Lithium carbonate	1000mg	Nocte	po
Imipramine	1000mg	MANE	po
Ibuprofen	400mg	BD	po
Zopiclone	150mg	Nocte	po
Haloperidol	15mg	TDS	po

22. An agitated patient

You are a thirty-two-year-old bachelor, who was diagnosed with schizophrenia eight years ago. Your mental health has been stable on olanzapine for the past five years, but you stopped taking your medication five months ago, because you felt you did not need it anymore. Since then you have felt increasingly suspicious and distressed. You are convinced that a group of drug dealers, about whom you complained to the local council, are targeting you. You know they are constantly watching you, and are trying to interfere with your thinking, by using their mobile phones. You have seen people driving slowly past your flat in black cars, looking at you in a threatening way.

You have phoned the police several times to complain about this surveillance, but they just ignore you. On the street, you have heard people making remarks such as: 'It's him', and 'He won't last'.

This morning, you punched a stranger, who was passing by in the street. He was talking on a mobile phone, and you are certain he was getting instructions to attack you.

The Police arrested you and took you to a nearby hospital. You are growing increasingly angry. You are finding it hard to control your voice, and occasionally shout out replies to questions. You are upset that they want you to see a psychiatrist. You don't think you are mentally ill, and you certainly don't need treatment. You want the Police to arrest the drug dealers.

During this interview, you will need to act as if you are agitated, clenching your fists and gesturing wildly. You will be angry with questioning initially, preferring to focus on those persecuting you. Gradually, you can start to calm down, and will answer questions more co-operatively.

23. Lower limb function

The actor is advised to act as normal. This station involves the candidate physically examining you.
Please follow any instructions given to you by the candidate.

24. Head injury

You are a sixty-five-year-old woman who was admitted to this psychiatric ward for treatment of your depression. You were started on antidepressant medication some days ago, but do not know what it is called. You have felt dizzy a few times since yesterday, when getting up abruptly from bed or standing up. You remember going to bed last night, but don't remember waking up or hitting your head. You are slightly confused and don't know the correct time, day or month. Initially, you keep your eyes closed, but open them when instructed to. You complain about a headache and a feeling of nausea. Please follow any instructions given by the candidate.

25. Apraxia, agnosia and Gerstmann's syndrome

You are a sixty-five-year-old man, who has had several small strokes affecting your brain in the last year. The candidate will ask you to do some tasks. You should demonstrate difficulties in writing, performing calculations, distinguishing left from right and recognizing your own fingers.
Please follow any instructions given to you by the candidate.

26. Korsakov's syndrome

You are a fifty-year-old man, who has been drinking alcohol to excess for many years. A while ago, you were admitted to hospital for a chest infection. Your memory is poor, but you are not aware of this. When prompted, reply that your memory is 'fine'.
Give incorrect answers to questions about where you are, and what time/day/ date/month/year it is.
When asked to remember words, you will be able to recall them immediately, but will make up words when asked to recall them a few minutes later. When asked about the names of the Prime Minister and the American President, please say 'Margaret Thatcher' and 'Ronald Reagan' respectively.

27. Cardiopulmonary resuscitation

A manikin is provided for this station.

28. Electroconvulsive (ECT) procedure

A manikin is provided for this station.

29. Language and non-dominant hemisphere functions

You are a forty-seven-year-old man, who has developed problems with naming things and understanding instructions, either written or spoken. When you speak, your sentences are short and simple.

Please follow any instructions given to you by the candidate.

15. Assessment for inpatient detention

In England and Wales, the relevant piece of law is Section 5 (2) of the Mental Health Act 1983, a holding power that enables a doctor to detain an inpatient in hospital for a further period of assessment of up to seventy-two hours. In other areas, it is expected that there will be some similar piece of legislation that permits detention of an inpatient against their will on the grounds of their health or safety or for the protection of others.

You would start by stating that you would have read through the patient's inpatient records, and have had a discussion with the nursing staff about their concerns, before interviewing the patient. It is also useful to state that you would interview the patient in a room that affords some privacy, with a member of staff present.

Introduces self.
Asks whether patient is aware of why he is being interviewed.
Explains the procedure of formal assessment under the Law.
Explains the possible outcomes.

Introduction |A| |B| |C| |D| |E|

Scene-setting |A| |B| |C| |D| |E|

⌘ Clarifies the details of the attempt to leave the ward.

⌘ Enquires about the reasons that prompted this. Asks whether he knows why the nurses stopped him from leaving.

Elicits reasons for attempt to leave |A| |B| |C| |D| |E|

Listening skills |A| |B| |C| |D| |E|

Rapport |A| |B| |C| |D| |E|

Empathy |A| |B| |C| |D| |E|

⌘ Reviews circumstances of admission.

⌘ Elicits details of the suicidal thoughts at the time. Had he made any plans?

⌘ Assesses current mental state:

- look for symptoms of depression, and biological symptoms
- look for prominent feelings of guilt and mood congruent delusions.

⌘ Enquires about suicidal thoughts or plans:

- how frequent are they? Has he thought about acting on them? Has he done anything so far? Had he made any plans? What was he intending to do when he left hospital?
- how much insight does he show into his own mental state?

⌘ Assesses level of risk.

Circumstances of admission	A	B	C	D	E

Current level of risk	A	B	C	D	E

⌘ Arrives at a decision regarding further detention in hospital:

- specify that the patient satisfies the legal criteria for detention in hospital
- informs patient of decision to continue detention and reasons for this
- specifies this is for a short period of time, to facilitate further assessment
- informs nursing staff
- it might be best to address the examiner and say that you would inform nursing staff of the decision, alert them to the suicidal thoughts expressed and agree the appropriate level of nursing observations. Say you would also fill out the relevant forms for the recommendation to detain the patient in hospital.

Factual knowledge	A	B	C	D	E

Informs patient	A	B	C	D	E

Informs staff	A	B	C	D	E

Ending	A	B	C	D	E

Global rating	A	B	C	D	E

This scenario can be continued in question 30, in which the findings can be discussed with a senior colleague.

16. Assessment of motivation to change

Introduces self.
Asks whether patient is aware of why he is being interviewed.

Introduction	A	B	C	D	E

⌘ Explores:

- reasons for giving up alcohol use, ie. physical health, mental health, occupation, relationships
- how circumstances have changed since last detoxification
- what plans have been made or actions taken to minimise relapse
- what he knows about anti-craving medications?
- what problems he expects during this critical period?
- what realistic goals has he planned?
- what support networks he has?

Listening skills   A B C D E

Empathy   A B C D E

⌘ Enquire about attempts to stop alcohol, both by himself and with help.

Careful attention should be paid to the measures taken by the patient to minimise the risk of lapse on this occasion, such as informing friends and other family members about his plans to give up alcohol, and requesting others not to offer him alcoholic drinks or beverages or avoiding drinking friends:

- ask about other plans taken by the patient to minimise lapse, such as, avoiding places associated with drinking cues such as pubs and off-licences
- ask about plans to attend voluntary agencies such as Alcoholics Anonymous (AA) or local relapse prevention groups.

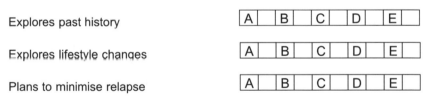

Explores past history   A B C D E

Explores lifestyle changes   A B C D E

Plans to minimise relapse   A B C D E

⌘ Explore short- and long-term goals:

- what does see himself doing in the absence of alcohol and drinking friends? What new hobbies or distraction techniques has he developed in order to keep himself away from alcohol?
- what realistic goals does he have?
- does he have the resources and support to achieve his goals?
- does he have a list of people or organisations to contact, should he have a lapse into drinking?

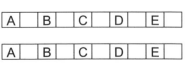

Explores goals   A B C D E

Ending   A B C D E

Global rating | A | | B | | C | | D | | E | |

17. Risk assessment in dementia

Introduces self.
Establishes rapport.
Is sensitive to daughter's concerns.

Communication | A | | B | | C | | D | | E | |

⌘ Obtains information about mother's current situation.

⌘ Enquires about daughter's concerns.

Assessment of current situation | A | | B | | C | | D | | E | |

⌘ Examines risks to self at home.

⌘ Assesses current mood state and suicidality.

⌘ Assess current mood state from what her daughter says:

- are there any symptoms or signs of depression?
- does she feel her life is worth living?
- has she mentioned suicide or not wanting to live?

Self-care and hygiene

- Is she looking after herself?
- Does she attend to her personal hygiene?
- Does she wash or take a bath?

Susceptibility to illness

- Is she physically well? Has she had any infections?
- Has she suffered from urinary tract infections? Would she recognize if she had a urinary tract infection?
- Has she had treatment for any physical complaint recently? Does she take her prescribed medication?

Food and fluid-intake

- Is she eating sufficiently?
- Does she drink enough?
- Can she tell whether food is stale or has gone off?

Mobility and falls

❖ Does she have any problems with mobility?
❖ Does she use a walking stick or frame?
❖ Has she had any falls? If so, did she sustain any injuries? Has she lost consciousness after a fall?
❖ Can she contact anyone in case of a fall? Does she have a panic alarm?
❖ Would she know what to do in case of an emergency?

Operating of equipment

❖ Is she able to operate the micro-wave oven safely?
❖ Is there a gas-stove? Does she use it? Has she ever left it on or unattended?

	A	B	C	D	E
Mood					
Self care and hygiene					
Susceptibility to physical illness					
Medication and alcohol					
Food and fluid intake					
Mobility and falls					
Safe operation of kitchen equipment					

⌘ Examines risks to self outside home and from others.

Wandering

❖ Is she aware of her environment?
❖ Does she usually know where she is?
❖ Has she ever lost her way? How did she get back home?
❖ Has she ever left the house at unusual times?

Vulnerability to abuse

❖ Is she safe at home?
❖ Could anyone take advantage of her financially or in other ways?
❖ Would she know if anyone tried to take advantage of her?

⌘ Examines risk to others:

● does she accept help from carers, either from the family or voluntary organisations?

- has she ever been threatening or aggressive?
- has she ever hit, kicked, scratched or bitten anyone?

Wandering | A | B | C | D | E |

Vulnerability to abuse | A | B | C | D | E |

Risk to others | A | B | C | D | E |

⌘ Discusses options to address the risks identified. Ask whether she has any questions about:

- making personal arrangements for her mother's care
- home-care, either from the local council or privately
- day centres
- residential homes
- nursing homes.

Risk management options | A | B | C | D | E |

Ending | A | B | C | D | E |

Global rating | A | B | C | D | E |

18. Bulimia nervosa

Introduces self, and explains reason for meeting with a psychiatrist:

> *Hello, Ms White. Your GP has asked me to see you because he is concerned about how you have been feeling lately, and especially as he thinks it may be in some way linked to your concerns about your physical health. Could we perhaps start by talking about how you have been feeling in yourself lately?*

> The key point to remember is that she may not understand why she needs to talk to a psychiatrist and she may not be too forthcoming if you launch into questions about her eating problems right at the beginning. Once you have established some rapport, you can ask more focused questions.

Introduction | A | B | C | D | E |

Establishes rapport | A | B | C | D | E |

Tactful questioning | A | B | C | D | E |

⌘ Ascertains whether the classical triad of persistent preoccupation with eating (and the resulting episodic overeating), inappropriate compensatory behaviours (such as inducing vomiting, abusing purgatives and/or diuretics, alternating starvation, misuse of enemas, or excessive exercise), and morbid fear of fatness (with a self-imposed weight threshold below her 'healthy' weight), are present:

> *How have you been eating lately? Have you had any problems controlling how much you eat, or how often? Have you felt as if you were losing control of your eating during a binge? How long have you had this problem?*
> *Have you been putting on or losing weight lately? Do you know what your current weight is?*
> *What is your ideal weight? How hard have you been trying to achieve it? Have you been scared of putting on any weight? Would you consider yourself 'fat'? How seriously has your self-esteem and confidence been affected by how you see yourself in the mirror?*
> *Have your periods been affected at all?*

⌘ Ascertains daily dietary intake:

> *Could you take me through an average day, listing what you might eat regularly and then what you might get through during the course of an average binge?*

Diagnostic criteria | A | B | C | D | E |

Factual knowledge | A | B | C | D | E |

⌘ Elicits what measures have been taken to lose weight:

> *What sorts of things have you been doing to keep your weight down?*
> *Have you been making yourself sick? How often?*
> *Have you been using laxatives or water pills, exercising more than usual, or trying to compensate by starving?*

⌘ Elicits associated mood and biological symptoms:

> *How has your mood been with all these changes in your weight? When your mood has been particularly low, have you had thoughts of wanting to end it all? Have you acted on any of these thoughts?*
> *How have you been sleeping? Has your concentration been affected? For example, have you been able to watch television or read the newspaper?*

Elicits weight control measures | A | B | C | D | E |

Explores comorbid symptoms | A | B | C | D | E |

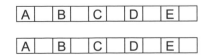

Physical complaints

- Diarrhoea, constipation, repeated urinary tract infections, history of seizures, lethargy, and hospitalization for electrolyte imbalance or renal impairment

Physical examination:

- Calculate current body mass index (BMI) $\frac{\text{weight in kgs}}{\text{height (in meters)}^2}$
- Head to toe examination focusing on the presence or not of dental erosion, bilateral parotid enlargement, peri-orbital oedema, calluses on the backs of hands (Russell's sign), tachy- and other arrhythmias, muscle weakness.

Elicits physical complaints	A	B	C	D	E
Explains procedure	A	B	C	D	E
Obtains consent	A	B	C	D	E
Performs relevant physical examination	A	B	C	D	E
Ending	A	B	C	D	E
Global rating	A	B	C	D	E

19. Management of acute dystonia

You may have actors representing the patient and/or nursing staff. The first task is to get a quick history (either directly from the actor representing the nurse or tell the examiner that you would like to talk to nursing staff beforehand to get relevant information).

You need to look at the patient's medical notes and prescription card. Make a note of the drugs he has had recently, and any dose changes or new drugs started. Specifically look for a history of illicit drug use.

Control of situation	A	B	C	D	E
Information from staff and notes	A	B	C	D	E

- State that the patient should be taken to a safe, private area, preferably a treatment room with emergency facilities.

- Ask if the patient can hear you, and whether he can respond.

- Reassure the patient. Explain that you will first examine him. Ask if you can proceed.

Ensure privacy | A | | B | | C | | D | | E | |

Reassure patient | A | | B | | C | | D | | E | |

Explain procedure and obtain verbal | A | | B | | C | | D | | E | |
consent

Rapid assessment of patient

❖ Check airway, breathing and circulation. If obviously dyspnoeic, request Nurse to arrange for bedside oxygen.

❖ Ask the nurse to take his pulse rate, blood pressure, and temperature while you:
- examine patient's tongue, eyes and neck (you can say out aloud that the patient shows signs of a focal dystonia with oculogyric crisis).

❖ Look for other relevant signs of extrapyramidal side-effects, such as limb rigidity.

Initial physical assessment | A | | B | | C | | D | | E | |

If your findings confirm a dystonic reaction, explain this to the patient briefly. The main points to mention are that it is known reaction to the medication and that he will be given an injection immediately to relieve his distress and pain. Inform the nurse present that this is a dystonic reaction and instruct the nurse to administer procyclidine 5–10 mg intramuscularly or intravenously (according to local protocol).

You should also mention that if the case was not as acute, and the patient could swallow, you might consider oral procyclidine. Alternatively, include benztropine and diazepam.

Explains finding to patient | A | | B | | C | | D | | E | |

Patient's concerns addressed | A | | B | | C | | D | | E | |

Immediate management | A | | B | | C | | D | | E | |

Instruct staff to monitor the patient's general condition and vital signs closely for the next forty-eight hours. If the patient has no relief of his symptoms within half an hour, they should alert you urgently.

You should also say that you will make a record of the episode in his notes, with details of your examination, immediate management and instructions for further management. You would also stop any antipsychotic medication, pending an urgent review by the treating team.

Further management | A | | B | | C | | D | | E | |

Documentation | A | | B | | C | | D | | E | |

Manner with nursing staff | A | | B | | C | | D | | E | |

Ending | A | | B | | C | | D | | E | |

Global rating | A | | B | | C | | D | | E | |

20. Rapid tranquillisation

You may have actors representing the patient and/or nursing staff. The first task is to get a quick history (either directly from the actor representing the nurse or tell the examiner that you would talk to nursing staff beforehand to get relevant information).

You need to look at the patient's medical notes (for diagnosis, Mental Health Act status, current treatment plan, and history of illicit drug use, and previous adverse reactions) and prescription card. Make a note of the drugs he has had recently, and any dose changes or new drugs instituted.

Specifically look for what medication he has had so far in this episode as well as over the previous twenty-four hours, and any recent depot medication.

⌘ What non-pharmacological techniques have been used so far?

History from staff and notes | A | | B | | C | | D | | E | |

Current medication and previous adverse effects | A | | B | | C | | D | | E | |

Medication used recently | A | | B | | C | | D | | E | |

Intervention used so far | A | | B | | C | | D | | E | |

If the scenario permits, try to interview the patient. Explain to him why he is being restrained and what will happen next.

It is usual to then follow one of the common algorithms for rapid tranquillisation, such as that advised by the Maudsley (Taylor *et al*, 2003). You should address this part to the examiner.

1. De-escalation, time out, placement techniques.
2. Offer oral treatment with either haloperidol 5mg or olanzapine 10mg or risperidone 1–2mg with or without lorazepam 1–2 mg; Repeat every forty-five to sixty minutes. Go to step 3 if three doses fail.
3. Consider haloperdol 5 mg im, or olanzapine 5–10 mg im, or ziprasidone 10–20 mg im, with or without lorazepam 1–2 mg im. Repeat up to three times at thirty-minute intervals, if insufficient effect. Promethazine 50 mg im is an alternative in benzodiazepine tolerant patients.
4. Consider intravenous treatment with diazepam 10 mg over at least five minutes. Repeat after five to ten minutes if insufficient effect (up to three times).
5. Seek expert advice.

Stepwise approach | A | | B | | C | | D | | E | |

Correct doses and routes |A| |B| |C| |D| |E| |

There are also several precautions, which you should elaborate on:

- Have flumazenil available to reverse the effects of lorazepam. Monitor respiratory rate and give flumazenil if respiratory rate falls below ten breaths per minute.
- Caution should be exercised in young and elderly.
- Ensure parental anticholinergic medication, such as procyclidine is available.
- It is preferable to use benzodiazepines and anti-psychotics in combination.
- Always confer with a senior colleague after a step of the algorithm is exhausted.
- Remember to consider the possibility of side-effects such as acute dystonia and NMS.
- Ensure close monitoring of vital signs.

Awareness of possible complications |A| |B| |C| |D| |E| |

Mentions relevant precautions |A| |B| |C| |D| |E| |

Post procedure monitoring |A| |B| |C| |D| |E| |

Considers personal safety and that of
others |A| |B| |C| |D| |E| |

Ending |A| |B| |C| |D| |E| |

Global rating |A| |B| |C| |D| |E| |

21. Drug interactions

Identifies the following:

1. Potential interaction between ibuprofen (NSAID) and lithium.
2. Doses of imipramine and zopiclone are above *BNF* limits.
3. Potential neurotoxicity between haloperidol and lithium.
4. Potential increase of lithium levels by approximately by 40% when prescribed with ibuprofen and other non-steroid anti-inflammatory drugs (NSAIDs).
5. Highlights the possibility of imipramine toxicity.

Identifies high doses |A| |B| |C| |D| |E| |

Identifies potential interactions |A| |B| |C| |D| |E| |

Stepwise approach |A| |B| |C| |D| |E| |

⌘ Discusses safer alternatives for analgesia such as aspirin or paracetamol.

⌘ Mentions review of patient's current notes for diagnosis, and management plan.

⌘ Mentions initial corrections to be made to the prescription card.

Practical tasks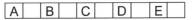

⌘ You must then address the clinical scenario.

⌘ Mention the differential diagnoses relevant to this presentation, namely lithium toxicity, and possibly serotonergic syndrome.

⌘ Briefly mention the initial steps in the management of lithium toxicity

Addresses clinical scenario | A | B | C | D | E |

Outlines initial management | A | B | C | D | E |

Ending | A | B | C | D | E |

Global rating | A | B | C | D | E |

(For further information see: Reimann *et al*, 1996; Cohen *et al*, 1974)

22. An agitated patient

Introduces self.
Explains the purpose of the interview.
Mentions the limited time available.
Mentions that there are staff nearby if any help is needed:

> *I have been asked to come and see you. I understand that the A&E staff are worried about you. I would like to ask you about what has been happening to you. I am afraid I'll have to be brief. The nursing staff will be available nearby if we need any assistance. Is that alright?*

Remains calm.
Establishes rapport.
Shows empathy.

Introduction | A | B | C | D | E |

Explanation | A | B | C | D | E |

Rapport | A | B | C | D | E |

Empathy | A | B | C | D | E |

- ❖ Starts by asking for patient's views of circumstances of his arrival.
- ❖ Uses open questions.
- ❖ Asks for clarification if in doubt.
- ❖ Structures the interview.
- ❖ Acknowledges patient's overt emotions.
- ❖ Non-confrontational interview style.

Question-framing | A | B | C | D | E | |

Acknowledges emotions | A | B | C | D | E | |

Structural interview | A | B | C | D | E | |

⌘ Obtains history of mental state in recent weeks:

> *When did you realize for the first time that something was wrong? How long has it been going on for? Who are the people persecuting you? How do you recognize them? Why would they target you? How convinced are you that this is really what is happening?*

Elicits recent mental state | A | B | C | D | E | |

⌘ Assesses risk:

> *Have you felt that you need to defend yourself against them? What happened today? Cold you tell me why you punched him? Is he part of the conspiracy? Did you feel under threat?*
> *Have you thought of harming anyone else? Have you made any plans?*
> *All of this must be distressing for you. Have you ever felt it was all too much to bear? Have you ever felt like ending your life? Have you made any plans?*

Risk assessment | A | B | C | D | E | |

⌘ Acknowledges the patient's distress.

⌘ Asks whether he would consider medication to help him with his distress.

⌘ Answer any questions that he may have.

⌘ Convey findings to nursing staff and give advice on appropriate medication.

Ending | A | B | C | D | E | |

Global rating | A | B | C | D | E | |

23. Lower limb function

Introduces self and explains purpose of the examination.
Gives clear instructions.
Is friendly and patient.
Obtains verbal consent.

Consent   A   B   C   D   E

Explanation   A   B   C   D   E

Use of language A   B   C   D   E

Tone

❖   Move hip, knee and ankle passively.

Power

❖   Test flexion and extension of the hip.
❖   Test abduction and adduction of the hip.
❖   Test flexion and extension of the knee.
❖   Test plantar flexion and dorsi-flexion of the ankle.

Tone and power   A   B   C   D   E

Tendon reflexes

❖   Test knee jerk.
❖   Test ankle jerk.
❖   Test plantar reflex: flexor response/extensor response (Babinski).

Reflexes   A   B   C   D   E

Sensation

❖   Test light touch.
❖   Test position sense.

Sensation   A   B   C   D   E

Coordination

❖   Test heel shin test.

Coordination   A   B   C   D   E

Gait

- ❖ Ask the patient to walk.
- ❖ Ask the patient to walk heel to toe on one line.
- ❖ Ask the patient to stand on one line.
- ❖ Test for pain.
- ❖ Test for weakness, eg. drop foot gait.
- ❖ Tests for spastic paralysis.
- ❖ Test for shuffling gait, rapid, small steps, absence of arm swinging (parkinsonism).
- ❖ Test for unsteadiness, wide base (cerebellar lesion, alcohol).

Gait

Interaction with patient

Ending

Global rating

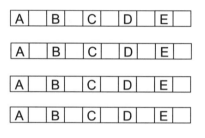

24. Head injury

Introduces self to any staff present and to the patient if she is conscious.
Addresses the patient.
Gives clear instructions.

Introduction

Communication

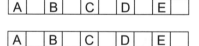

⌘ Assesses level of consciousness using the Glasgow Coma Scale (Teasdale and Jennet, 1974):

Checks whether patient opens eyes	
spontaneously	4
to verbal stimuli	3
to pain	2
never	I
Checks best verbal response	
orientated and converses	5
disorientated and converses	4
inappropriate words	3
incomprehensible sounds	2
none	I
Checks best motor response	
patient obeys	6
patient localizes pain	5
flexion withdrawal	4
flexion	3
extension	2
none	I

Level of consciousness   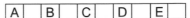 |A| |B| |C| |D| |E| |

⌘ Asks whether the patient remembers what happened.

⌘ Enquires what she remembers prior to the fall.

⌘ Enquires about physical symptoms:

- headache
- nausea
- vomiting
- dizziness
- blurred or double vision.

Common symptoms |A| |B| |C| |D| |E| |

⌘ Assesses cognitive functioning:

- orientation in time and place
- registration
- attention
- recall
- retrograde amnesia.

Orientation and memory |A| |B| |C| |D| |E| |

⌘ Performs relevant physical examination:

- pupillary reaction to light, consensual light reflex and reaction to accommodation
- injuries of scalp, head and neck
- bleeding or cerebro-spinal fluid from nose or ears
- focal neurological deficits
- other injuries.

Physical examination |A| |B| |C| |D| |E| |

⌘ Considers sub-dural haematoma or chronic sub-dural haematoma.

⌘ Mentions need for referral to A&E department for further assessment and observation.

⌘ Suggests appropriate level of observation while awaiting further assessment.

⌘ Suggests analgesia, such as paracetamol.

Explains need for further assessment |A| |B| |C| |D| |E| |

Ending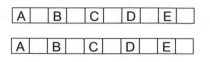

Global rating

25. Apraxia, agnosia and Gerstmann's syndrome

Introduces self.
Explains purpose of the examination.
Gives clear instructions.
Is patient throughout testing.

Explanation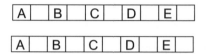

Communication and general manner

Apraxia

⌘ Asks patient to demonstrate how to:

- perform a salute
- stop traffic
- turn a key
- make a phone call
- brush his teeth
- use scissors.

⌘ Asks patient to copy interviewers own actions.

Apraxia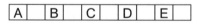

Agnosia

⌘ Asks patient to identify objects.

Agnosia

Asomatagnosia

⌘ Asks patient to identify body parts:

What do you call this part of your body?
Can you show me your hand, knee, wrist, elbow, or calf ?

Can you show me your left hand?

Colour agnosia

⌘ Asks patients to identify colours of objects.

Asomatagnosia and colour agnosia | A | | B | | C | | D | | E | |

Dysgraphesthesia

⌘ Instructs patient to close his eyes.

⌘ Asks patient to identify letters written on his palm with a pen-like object.

Astereognosis

⌘ Instructs patient to close his eyes.

⌘ Asks patient to identify objects like a coin, key, paperclip, or pen.

⌘ First in one hand then in the other.

Dysgraphesthesia and astereognosis | A | | B | | C | | D | | E | |

Gerstmann's syndrome

Agraphia/dysgraphia

⌘ Spontaneous writing:

  • Asks patient to write one or a few sentences on any topic

⌘ Dictation:

  • Asks patient to write down words like 'flame,' 'candle,' 'height,' and 'steak'.

Agraphia | A | | B | | C | | D | | E | |

Acalculia

⌘ Asks patient to write down numbers.

⌘ Asks patient to perform a simple addition, subtraction, multiplication, division tasks.

⌘ Asks patient to perform more complex calculations.

Acalculia |A| |B| |C| |D| |E| |

Left-right disorientation

Can you show me your right hand?
Can you point to your left ear?
Can you touch your right ear with your left hand?
Which is my left hand?

Left-right disorientation |A| |B| |C| |D| |E| |

Finger agnosia

Which finger did I just touch?
Can you move your middle finger?
Can you name this finger on my hand?

Finger agnosia |A| |B| |C| |D| |E| |

Ending |A| |B| |C| |D| |E| |

Global rating |A| |B| |C| |D| |E| |

26. Korsakov's syndrome

Introduces self.
Establishes rapport.
Is patient and sensitive to the patient's difficulties.
Introduces the tests and explains the procedure clearly.

Communications |A| |B| |C| |D| |E| |

Explanation |A| |B| |C| |D| |E| |

Introductory questions

⌘ Asks questions like:

How is your memory in general?
Are you able to remember things?
Have you been more forgetful lately?
Have you forgotten appointments lately?

Introductory questions |A| |B| |C| |D| |E| |

⌘ Assesses orientation:

- Orientation in time:
  ~ asks for the year, season, day, date and month
  ~ asks additional questions: 'What is the time of day?', 'How long have you been here?', and 'How long have we been speaking?'
- Orientation in place:
  ~ asks for the country, county, town/village, address or building, floor/ward
  ~ asks additional questions: 'What kind of building are we in?'

Orientation |A| |B| |C| |D| |E| |

Assesses short-term memory

⌘ Registration:

- gives three unrelated words and asks to repeat these words
- prompts the patient to remember the words, as they will be asked again
  or
- asks the patient to remember a name and address, eg. Peter Brown, 42 Church Lane, Southampton
- prompts the patient to remember the address, as it will be asked again.

Registration |A| |B| |C| |D| |E| |

⌘ Attention/distraction:

- gives patient a task to test attention and to distract him prior to testing for recall, ie. asking him to spell the word 'world' backwards or asking him to recite the months of the year backwards from December.

⌘ Recall:

- asks whether the patient can recall any of the three words he was asked to remember earlier on
  or
- asks whether the patient can recall the name and address he was asked to remember earlier on.

Recall |A| |B| |C| |D| |E| |

Assesses long-term memory

Do you read a newspaper or watch the news on TV?
Can you recall anything in the news that has caught your interest?
Do you watch sports? Which match was on recently? Who won? **or** *What was the result?*

What is the name of the Prime Minister?
Who was the previous Prime Minister?
What is the name of the American President?

Long-term memory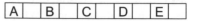

❊ Checks for confabulation — this may have been evident from some of the previous answers. If not, it may be useful to ask the patient questions about what they had done that day or what meal they had that morning. Explain to the examiner that you would need to confirm what was said with nursing staff or carer.

❊ Checks for perseveration — this repetition of words, phrases or questions would also be evident during the interview.

Confabulation/perseveration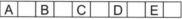

❊ Explains need for further investigations and tests.

❊ Asks whether the patient has any questions.

Ending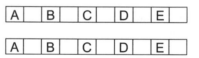

Global rating

27. Cardiopulmonary resuscitation (CPR)

As this station has a manikin representing the patient, you will have to say out aloud what you are looking for or doing. To fully demonstrate the procedure, always proceed as if this is a worst case scenario, ie. not breathing and pulseless.

❊ Initial approach:

❖ Check that you can approach safely (rescuer safety).
❖ When you are next to the patient, look for a response. This is usually done by 'shaking and shouting.' So, first, shout out 'Hello, hello, can you hear me?' Give him a command, 'Open your eyes!' Shake him by his shoulders. Say you have not had a response and proceed.
❖ Check his mouth (for any obvious obstruction, like dislodged dentures).
❖ Open the airway, by tilting his head.
❖ Check his breathing for ten seconds. (Lean forward and **look** for his chest moving. At the same time, **listen** for sounds of breathing, and **feel** his breath against your cheek). Say that he is not breathing and proceed.
❖ You are now supposed to go for help. If you alone and you could tell the person was in this condition due to injury, drowning or is an infant or child, say that you would perform resuscitation for one minute before seeking help. As the scenario is based on a ward, you should probably say you will check the rest of the crash team

has been called or that an ambulance has been called for. When demonstrating, pretend to point to someone and say clearly, 'Please call for an ambulance, and report back'.

Initial approach |A| |B| |C| |D| |E|

Explanation of each step |A| |B| |C| |D| |E|

Check for breathing |A| |B| |C| |D| |E|

Gets help |A| |B| |C| |D| |E|

Cardiopulmonary resuscitation procedure:

❖ Give two breaths (make sure you squeeze (seal) his nose and make a proper seal with your mouth).
❖ Check for signs of circulation (classically we are taught to look for a pulse, but in the heat of the moment mistakes can happen, so it is now convention to look for the person's colour, and for any spontaneous movement). Say you have not found any signs of circulation.
❖ Commence chest compressions. Feel his sternum, and locate the lower end. Position your hands, one on top of the other, about two finger breaths away from the lower sternal notch. Keep your elbows straight. Depress the chest wall for at least a third of the way down and release. You need to do them at the rate of 100 per minute. Perform fifteen compressions and then give two breaths. Repeat the cycle. State that you won't stop until help arrives, or the patient moves or takes a spontaneous breath.
❖ It is also useful to state that if at any stage you detect breathing or a circulation, you will turn the patient into the recovery position (you should be able to describe this position).

Gives effective breaths |A| |B| |C| |D| |E|

Checks for circulation |A| |B| |C| |D| |E|

Effective chest compressions |A| |B| |C| |D| |E|

Repeat cycle correctly |A| |B| |C| |D| |E|

Ending |A| |B| |C| |D| |E|

Global rating |A| |B| |C| |D| |E|

For further information see: Resuscitation Council, 2000; Handley *et al*, 2001. In addition, most NHS trusts have their own local resuscitation guidelines.

28. Electroconvulsive therapy (ECT) procedure

As this station has a manikin representing the patient, some of the conversation may be addressed to the examiner.

You may start by asking for the patient's notes. Say that you would look for the entry from the team doctor where this session of ECT is prescribed. You would look for medication the patient is on and confirm the exact doses of all medication taken in the last twenty-four hours, looking especially for any drugs that might raise the seizure threshold (eg. benzodiazepines) or lower it (eg. antipsychotics). You would confirm with nursing staff that the patient has not had food for at least eight hours before, and that the patient has voided just prior to entering the treatment room. You would also confirm that informed consent has been obtained and that it has been clearly documented in the notes. Introduce yourself to the patient and ask again for verbal consent for this episode of treatment. As there is only a limited amount of time for the entire OSCE task, you may want to summarise what you would say to the patient:

> *I would explain the actual procedure, and expected benefits and potential side-effects both of the treatment itself and of general anaesthesia. I would then ask the patient if he has understood what I have said, ask him to tell me in his own words what he has understood and answer any questions he might have. I would then ask if he consents to this administration of ECT, reassure him that he may withdraw consent at any time and document his response in the notes.*

The key point is to ask for consent again, just prior to the treatment but without any undue pressure, and to document it.

Introduction

A	B	C	D	E

Checks medical notes, prescription order and consent

A	B	C	D	E

Obtains consent and records it

A	B	C	D	E

Pre-treatment procedure:

❖ Check that all the relevant equipment is in place. Say out aloud that you will look for the ECT machine, electrodes, gel, and resuscitation equipment. Say that you would expect that all equipment had been checked but that you will confirm that nothing is missing or obviously defective.

❖ Decide on the dose to be administered for this treatment, and adjust the ECT machine accordingly. (In practice, you will use the lowest possible dose according to the charts for the machine, and taking into account the patient's age, sex, medication, and previous treatment record and then gradually increase the dose according to whether an adequate seizure occurs. This process is called 'stimulus dosing' and an 'adequate' motor seizure is thought to be one that lasts at least fifteen seconds (Royal College of Psychiatrists, 1995). Check that all restrictive clothing and dentures are removed. Check that there is a watch/clock available to time the seizure (some machines may have an inbuilt EEG that accurately records when the seizure begins and ends).

Pre-treatment checks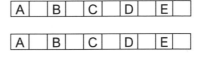

Dose determination

Treatment procedure

❖ Confirm with the anaesthetist that the procedure for general anaesthesia can begin. Usually, the anaesthetist will establish an intravenous line and administer an anaesthetic and muscle relaxant. You can say that while this is being done, you will check the electrodes, and pour contact gel onto them. Once the patient is unconscious, you can clean the sites where you are going to place the electrodes. Current practice is to use bilateral electrode placements (Royal College of Psychiatrists, 1995). For this, electrodes should be placed frontotemporally 4 cm above the midpoint of an imaginary line between the tragus and the external canthus. If describing unilateral ECT, one electrode is placed at the right frontotemporal position, the other 4 cm inferior to the midpoint of a line joining the right and left tragus in a coronal plane on the right side of the head.

❖ Ensure that you hold the electrodes with your thumbs over the trigger button and the ulnar edges of your hands facing inwards, so that you are gently pressing inwards at the electrode sites. If the test or trigger buttons are not on the electrodes, but are elsewhere on the machine, confirm with a nursing colleague that they are willing to press them at your command. Check they know which is for testing and which for the actual current administration.

Initial treatment procedure

Electrode placement

❖ Confirm with the anaesthetist whether you can proceed. Administer a test dose to check electrode placement and whether adequate contact is made. If so, say out aloud a warning (usually the word 'clear') and administer the current. Say that you are will watch for the seizure to be evident, (usually starting as a slight tremor in the extremities) and that you will time it from beginning to end. Say that if it is not of adequate duration, you will consider a second administration, at a higher dose, and only once you have asked the anaesthetist if you can do so.

❖ In practice, you should go on as if the seizure was adequate during this OSCE, unless told by the examiner otherwise. Confirm to the anaesthetist that the treatment has been completed.

Test dose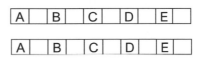

Actual dose administration

Timing of seizure duration | A | | B | | C | | D | | E | |

Post treatment procedure:

❖ Watch the patient carefully as the anaesthetist brings the patient out of anaesthesia. Usually, this ends with the anaesthetist asking the patient to confirm his name. Say that you will be particularly watching out for post-seizure delirium (in which the patient may thrash about and appear confused, and which is managed by reassurance, calmly talking to and gently moving the patient).

❖ Say that you will turn the patient into the recovery position and ensure that all monitors are correctly working as the patient is shifted to the recovery room. Say that the patient will have frequent observations recorded over the next hour or so whilst in the recovery room, which would be done by the assigned nurse. You will stay for the entire period of recovery, ensuring that the patient is comfortable and providing reassurance where necessary. You will also record the details of the treatment, including dose administered, duration of seizure, any complications and remarks the recovery period. You may need to countersign the anaesthetist's notes of the treatment and recovery period.

Post-treatment disorder | A | | B | | C | | D | | E | |

Ending | A | | B | | C | | D | | E | |

Global rating | A | | B | | C | | D | | E | |

29. Language and non-dominant hemisphere functions

Introduces self.
Establishes rapport.
Gives clear instructions.
Is sensitive to patients difficulties.

Communication | A | | B | | C | | D | | E | |

⌘ Tests aphasia/dysphasia.

⌘ Tests spontaneous language, eg. by asking about work or family.

⌘ Examines naming:

   • asks names of every day objects like pen, watch, button, etc
   • asks less familiar objects like strap, buckle, winder, collar, sleeve.

Spontaneous language | A | | B | | C | | D | | E | |

Naming | A | | B | | C | | D | | E | |

⌘ Examines comprehension.

⌘ Uses common objects like pen, key, coin, watch or chair:

- ask the patient to point at different objects in turn
- ask the patient to point at less familiar objects
- give commands to test verbal comprehension, such as: 'Touch the watch with the pen' or 'put the keys under the chair'.

What object is used to open a door? Which one is for writing?
Is my wife's husband a man or a woman?
What instrument would you use to cut wood? What would you use to light a fire?

Comprehension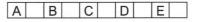

⌘ Examines repetition:

- asks patient to repeat simple words like 'pen,' 'clock,' 'house', etc
- asks patient to repeat more complex words, such as 'hospital,' 'politics,' 'basketball player', etc
- asks patient to repeat complex sentences, such as, 'don't bury your head in the sand', 'the quick brown fox jumped over the lazy dog' or 'no ifs, ands or buts'.

Repetition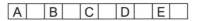

⌘ Tests alexia/dyslexia:

- letter identification
- asks patient to name individual letters.

Reading aloud

❖ Asks patient to read words, sentences or a short paragraph out aloud.

Comprehension

❖ Gives a written command, eg. close your eyes and asks patient to follow the command.
❖ Gives patient a paragraph to read and asks him to explain its meaning.

Dyslexia

A	B	C	D	E

⌘ Tests non-dominant hemisphere function.

Hemi-neglect

⌘ Assesses hemi-neglect by testing:

- sensation on both sides
- visual fields
- extinction when stimulation is offered on both sides simultaneously.

Hemi-neglect | A | | B | | C | | D | | E | |

Hemi-spatial neglect

⌘ Asks patient to:

- draw a face, house or clock-face
- copy a two-headed flower
- bisect a line.

Hemi-spatial neglect | A | | B | | C | | D | | E | |

Constructional apraxia

⌘ Asks the patient to draw:

- a house
- intersecting pentagons
- a three-dimensional shape like a cube.

Constructional apraxia | A | | B | | C | | D | | E | |

Ending | A | | B | | C | | D | | E | |

Global rating | A | | B | | C | | D | | E | |

References

Cohen R *et al* (1974) Lithium carbonate, haloperidol and irreversible brain damage. *JAMA* **230**: 1283–7

Handley A, Monsieurs K, Bossaert L (2001) ERC Guidelines for Adult Basic Life Support. *Resuscitation* **48**: 199–205. Online at: www.erc.edu

Reimann *et al* (1996) Indomethacin but not aspirin increases plasma lithium ion levels. *Arch Gen Psychiatry* **143**: 882–4

The Royal College of Psychiatrists (1995) *The ECT handbook. Council Report CR39*. Royal College of Psychiatrists, London

Resuscitation Council UK (2000) Resuscitation Guidelines. Online at: www.resus.org.uk

Taylor D *et al* (2003) *The South London and Maudsley NHS 2003 Prescribing Guidelines*. 7th edn. Martin Dunitz, London

Teasdale G, Jennet B (1974) Assessment of coma and impaired consciousness: a practical scale. *Lancet* 13: 18–83

Section three:
Communications skills

30. Discussion with senior colleague (this can be practised as the station that follows question 15)

You have just assessed a twenty-two-year-old man on a psychiatric ward. He had been stopped from leaving by nursing staff, who were concerned at his mental state. On assessment, he is severely depressed, with delusions of guilt. He is suicidal, and wants to be allowed home to make a serious attempt on his life.

Discuss your findings with the duty specialist registrar/consultant over the telephone.

31. Explanation of diagnosis: borderline personality disorder

The mother of a twenty-six-year-old patient would like to speak with you. Her daughter is about to be discharged from hospital after her nineteenth inpatient admission. At the discharge care programme approach (CPA) meeting, they were told that she has a diagnosis of 'borderline personality disorder', and she want to know what this means.

She lives alone and is unemployed. Her two children, now aged three and five, are in foster care. She has been harming herself since her late teens, by taking overdoses of medication, or cutting her wrists. On one occasion, three years ago, she tried to hang herself. These episodes have always occurred when she has been feeling distressed or particularly 'emotional'. Most of the time though, she complains of feeling 'empty' or bored. She has distressing mood swings on most days, which can result in outbursts of anger, when she lashes out at anyone or anything nearby.

She tends to live her life recklessly, drifting from one relationship to another and bingeing on alcohol and illicit drugs. She does not trust people but has no difficulty forming sexual relationships with both men and women. She has only recently told you that she was sexually and physically abused as a child, by various foster fathers.

32. Explanation of side-effects: antipsychotics

This twenty-three-year-old lady, currently on olanzapine 10mg daily, is worried about the possible side-effects of anti-psychotic medications.

Explore her concerns and explain the side effects of this medication.

33. Management of weight gain

This twenty-four-year-old man has noticed his weight increasing gradually over the past fourteen months. He is on olanzapine 15mg daily and attends your outpatient clinic. He has been compliant with his medication and appreciates the need to be on it.

Advise him on weight management.

34. Explanation of action: antipsychotics

The next patient in your outpatient clinic is on treatment with risperidone 4mg daily, for schizophrenia. She would like more about her medication.

Explain the mechanism of action and side-effects of her medication.

35. Explanation of cognitive therapy for depression

This patient is a forty-five-year-old with a history of mild depression for the last four years. She has been tried on three different classes of antidepressant, at appropriate doses and for adequate lengths of time, without much effect. You would now like to consider a referral for cognitive therapy.

Assess this patient for and explain cognitive therapy to her.

36. Explanation of diagnosis: schizophrenia

This twenty-year-old man was admitted to hospital a month ago. He was convinced at the time of admission that he was under surveillance by MI5. He could hear people's voices coming out of microphones in the walls of his house. After treatment with antipsychotic medication, his psychosis abated, and he is now ready for discharge. He would like to know more about his diagnosis of schizophrenia.

Explain the diagnosis of schizophrenia to him.

37. Breaking bad news

This fifty-four-year-old male patient is being treated on your ward for depression. You have just been informed by a staff nurse that staff at a nearby medical ward called to say that his wife, who was terminally ill after poorly responding to renal dialysis for chronic renal failure, passed away ten minutes ago.

Inform the patient of his wife's death.

38. Discontinuation of lithium

This fifty-year-old lady has been referred to your out patient clinic by her GP. She would like to come off lithium tablets, a medication she has been on for many years.

Assess the presentation and advise accordingly.

39. Explanation of vascular dementia

The wife of a seventy-two-year-old patient has asked to see you. She would like to ask you some questions about her husband, who has recently been diagnosed with vascular dementia.

Discuss vascular dementia with the carer.

40. Explanation of psychodynamic psychotherapy

You have been asked to speak to this thirty-five-year-old woman who has recently been referred for individual psychodynamic therapy for low self-esteem and relationship difficulties. She is currently on the waiting-list and has asked to speak to somebody because she has some questions that she would like to ask.

Explore the presentation and address any questions or concerns she may have.

41. Referral of a confused patient to a medical colleague

Last night a seventy-year-old woman was admitted to your psychiatric ward. She presented with confusion and delusional ideas. She had told her eighty-year-old husband that people had entered their flat, and were trying to kill her.

She has no previous psychiatric history and has not been confused before. She has had two transient ischaemic attacks (TIAs) in the last six months. She is on propanolol to treat her hypertension.

The first night on the ward she was anxious and restless. She appeared vacant and at times seemed to respond to visual hallucinations. Her speech was incoherent and she was disorientated for time and place. She kept asking for her husband repeatedly.

In the morning she seemed slightly more alert and orientated.

On physical examination her temperature was 37.5° C and she had some lower abdominal tenderness.

A routine blood-test was done on admission which showed a white cell count of 14.3×10^9/litre and an ESR of 20 mm/hr. Her sodium was 129mmol/l. A midstream urine speciman (MSU) showed the protein level to be '++.'

You suspect the patient is suffering from delirium and decide to refer her for a medical assessment.

Contact the medical SHO on the telephone and refer the patient for a medical opinion.

42. Agoraphobia and behavioural therapy

Ms B is a thirty-five-year-old single lady, who has been referred to your outpatient clinic by her GP. She has been housebound for the last year, as she becomes anxious when around crowds or on public transport. She had a panic attack last month, and is now even more unwilling to leave home for fear of having another attack. She was started on an antidepressant six weeks ago, but her GP thinks she may also benefit from behavioural therapy.

Assess the extent that her symptoms disable her day-to-day functioning and explain behavioural therapy to her.

43. Lithium in pregnancy

This thirty-five-year-old lady, with a five year history of bipolar affective disorder and several inpatient admissions, has asked to see you in the outpatient clinic. Most of her previous depressive relapses have necessitated Mental Health Act detention in view of the risk of suicide, and have resulted in extreme disruption to her social and occupational functioning. Her GP told her that she was pregnant yesterday, and she has asked for this urgent appointment because she is on lithium therapy.

Address her concerns and discuss lithium therapy in pregnancy.

44. Discharge plans

This forty-five-year-old man was admitted under Mental Health Act detention to your hospital for treatment of an acute psychotic episode. His psychosis has been treated over the last four months, initially with oral and then later, depot antipsychotic medication, due to initial non-compliance. He is being discharged from hospital today, and your consultant has asked you to discuss the discharge care plan with the patient. Your notes of the pre-discharge care programme approach meeting state:

'Discharge plans:
~ Outpatient follow-up by SHO at CMHT
~ Regular mental health reviews by CPN
~ Continue on depot fluphenazinedecanoate 100mg im, two-weekly, to be administered at depot clinic
~ Patient has contact number for the crisis team
~ Next CPA meeting 14 April
~ Enhanced level CPA, CPN will be care co-ordinator'.

Discuss the discharge plan and aftercare arrangements with the patient.

45. Compliance

This forty-five-year-old man, with a ten-year history of schizophrenia, is about to be discharged from hospital after his fifth admission. He has relapsed on all previous occasions due to abruptly stopping his medication of his own accord.

Explore his compliance with treatment and discuss interventions that may help him in the future.

Instructions for actors

30. Discussion with senior colleague

It is expected that for this OSCE, the actor would in fact have to be an examiner, or a psychiatric colleague.

You are the duty senior psychiatrist. You are about to receive a phone call from the duty senior house officer in psychiatry. He/she has just assessed an inpatient and would like to discuss the case with you. The salient features are that the twenty-two-year old man is severely depressed with delusions of guilt. He is acutely suicidal, and was attempting to leave the ward to commit suicide when he was stopped by nursing staff, and detained under nurses' emergency holding powers.

31. Explanation of diagnosis: borderline personality disorder

You are the step-mother of a twenty-six-year-old lady, who is about to be discharged from a psychiatric hospital following her nineteenth inpatient admission after taking an overdose of paracetamol. You have asked to speak to the doctor today because you were told at the discharge planning meeting that she has a 'borderline personality disorder', and you want to know what that means and how you can help her in future.

She lives alone and is unemployed. Her two children, now aged three and five, are in foster care. She has been harming herself since her late teens, by taking overdoses of medication, or cutting her wrists. On one occasion, three years ago, she tried to hang herself. These episodes have always occurred when she has been feeling distressed or particularly 'emotional'. Most of the time though, she complains of feeling empty or bored. She has distressing mood swings on most days, which can result in outbursts of anger, when she lashes out at anyone or anything nearby.

She tends to live her life recklessly, drifting from one relationship to another and bingeing on alcohol and illicit drugs. She does not trust people but has no difficulty forming sexual relationships with both men and women. She has only recently told you that she was sexually and physically abused as a child, by various foster fathers.

32. Explanation of side-effects: antipsychotics

You are a twenty-three-year-old lady, who has been on a medication called olanzapine at a dose of 10mg daily for the past two months. Over the past two years, you have felt suspicious of others and 'paranoid' about your safety. It all seems to have begun after you had a bad experience with amphetamines.

You now feel well on this medication. You attend the local mental health resource centre as a day patient. The other day you spoke to a fellow patient, who spoke of many different and worrying side-effects that she had found out about on the internet. The ones you are most concerned about include not being able to have children and the possibility of having abnormal movements and even a heart attack. Although you remember some of these side-effects being explained to you before you started the tablets, you'd like to speak with a doctor about them again.

33. Management of weight gain

You are a twenty-four-year-old man, who suffered a psychotic breakdown about a year ago. You recovered with the help of medication and have not heard voices or felt any paranoia since your initial admission. You are now working and have a girlfriend. You have noticed a gain in weight of about 9 kg since you started the medication you are on, which is called olanzapine. Your family and girlfriend have commented on your weight and you would like advice from the doctor about the weight problem.

You smoke fifteen cigarettes daily, and tend to binge-drink over weekends. You might drink up to twenty cans of lager over a weekend. Most of your meals are take-aways or from fast food outlets. You stopped playing football a few weeks before you first became ill, and now are not physically active at all.

34. Explanation of action: antipsychotics

You are a twenty-eight-year-old lady, who has been in a stable relationship for the last year. You were admitted to hospital eighteen months ago, after several months of hearing voices and believing you were under surveillance by the security services. Whilst in hospital, you were started on a medication called Risperidone. It helped to reduce the intensity of the voices and made you gradually less paranoid. Unfortunately, you have also put on a few kilos in weight since your hospitalisation. This has caused you a lot of concern, and you are now unsure about whether to continue on the medication or not. You have not heard voices for over a month. On the internet, you read that schizophrenia is caused by a chemical imbalance in the brain. You would like to know more from the doctor.

35. Explanation of cognitive therapy for depression

You are a forty-five-year-old accountant. For the last four years, you have been depressed. You are constantly tired, and find it difficult to concentrate at work. You are always critical of yourself and feel you could be accomplishing more with your life. Your psychiatrists have tried to treat the depression with three different drugs. However, you have not benefited from any of them. You have heard from friends that some people with depression are treated with cognitive therapy, and you would like to know more.

36. Explanation of diagnosis: schizophrenia

You are a twenty-year-old man, who was admitted to hospital a month ago. You were convinced at the time of admission that you were under surveillance by MI5. You could hear people's voices coming out of microphones in the walls of your house. After treatment with oral medication, these symptoms became much less intrusive, and you are now ready for discharge. You would like to get back to work, but aren't sure if that is advisable. You would like to know more about your diagnosis of schizophrenia, and especially what to do to avoid future breakdowns.

37. Breaking bad news

You are a fifty-four-year-old man, who has been treated on this psychiatric ward for depression over the last three weeks. Your wife was admitted at around the same time, to the local dialysis unit, as she needed urgent treatment for kidney failure. You last spoke with her yesterday, and visited her two days ago. Her doctors had been worried that she was not responding to the treatment. Your mood had been worse since your last visit to see her.

You have not anticipated her death and have not made any preparations for it. The last time you were asked about it, you refused to talk to the nurses about her ill health.

This doctor will break the sad news of your wife's death to you. You will initially feel numb, and will respond to questions slowly. Then you will become distressed and deny that it has happened. You will ask for proof. After a while, you will start becoming angry at her doctors and blame them for her death. You will be tearful and will shout out aloud at times.

38. Discontinuation of lithium

You are a fifty-year-old secretary who lives at home with her solicitor husband. You have suffered from manic depression for most of your life, and had several hospital admissions in early adulthood. Your last spell in hospital, about sixteen years ago, occurred after you tried to stop Lithium of your own accord. For the last fourteen years however, you have been well, and have been seen only by your GP for repeat prescriptions of Lithium, and the occasional blood test. You have always taken 800 milligrams of lithium at night. Although you have a mild tremor of the hands, you have never noticed any other side-effects with this medication. Whilst looking at the internet recently, you found out that lithium has been known to cause serious side-effects including failure of the kidneys, and the thyroid gland. You also learnt that there are newer medications that do not cause these side effects. You have come to this appointment to discuss treatment options and to help you decide whether or not to continue on lithium . You are particularly concerned about the risk of becoming ill again.

39. Explanation of vascular dementia

Your husband, who is seventy-two years old, has recently been diagnosed with vascular dementia. He also suffers from diabetes, which is controlled with a tablet called Metformin. He smokes ten cigarettes a day. He had a heart-attack two years ago and has had funny turns several times. On one occasion he collapsed and couldn't use his right hand for a while. On another occasion he couldn't speak for a few hours.

Over the last year he has become increasingly confused. His illness seems to get worse in stages. At times he can be restless and agitated. He also has become rather clumsy and is not looking after his personal hygiene. He seems confused about which way around he should wear his clothes. You have written down the questions you would like to ask the doctor:

What is vascular dementia?
What causes it?
Is it different from Alzheimer's?
Can anything be done about it?
What can I expect in the future?
What kind of help will be available when I am struggling?

40. Explanation of psychodynamic psychotherapy

You are a thirty-five-year-old woman. You recently had a psychiatric outpatient appointment for chronic feelings of low self-esteem and difficulties in your relationships with men. You have been referred for psychodynamic therapy and are currently on the waiting-list.

You have asked to speak to somebody, because you are slightly weary and have some questions that you would like to ask:

What is psychotherapy?
What can I expect from the therapist?
What is the procedure of the therapy?
Does it help?

41. Referral of a confused patient to a medical colleague

You are the medical SHO in the local district hospital, which is four miles away from the mental health unit. You have been telephoned by the psychiatric SHO, who asks for a medical assessment on a seventy-year-old woman, who was admitted to the psychiatric ward last night with confusion and paranoid ideas. You are not convinced she needs a medical opinion and need a lot of persuasion to agree to the request. Your main reason for this reluctance is that you think that she is just psychotic or dementing.

42. Agoraphobia and behavioural therapy

You are a thirty-five-year-old single lady, who works in a bank. You have been off sick from work since your relationship with your ex-boyfriend ended over a year ago. As you had common friends, you began avoiding social occasions. Over time, you noticed that you became increasingly fearful of going out at all. Last month, you decided to go out with your one close friend. Unfortunately, you became extremely anxious because you felt you were surrounded by too many people. You thought you were going to die or have a heart attack. You started shaking, and sweating and had to rush back home. Your GP says that you had a panic attack, and he has started you on an antidepressant. Although your mood has lifted a bit, you are still mostly housebound. You do all of your shopping on the internet, and only go out for appointments with your doctor. Your mother does any tasks that might require you to go out. Your fear now extends to being alone in open spaces, as well as on the buses and trains. You are keen to get back to work as soon as possible, but can't see a way forward because of your fear of going out and using public transport.

43. Lithium in pregnancy

You are a thirty-five-year-old actress with a five year history of manic depression. When you have been ill in the past, your mood has been either extremely depressed (and suicidal) or elated ('high'), and you have invariably needed hospitalisation for up to several months. During these relapses of your illness, you have lost work, and have alienated your family and friends, and it has always taken a long time to get back to your former life. For the last two years however, your mood has been stable on therapy with lithium tablets, and you have re-established your career and relationships. You have asked for this urgent appointment with the psychiatrist because you found out yesterday that you're pregnant, and you think you may have been warned about becoming pregnant on lithium therapy.

44. Discharge plans

You are a forty-five-year-old bus driver, who was admitted to hospital four months ago after what was termed an 'acute psychotic breakdown.' You tried to punch a stranger on your bus in response to voices that you'd been hearing in your head. In hospital, you have been treated with tablets which you only pretended to take, and then, when you were found out, with an injection once every two weeks. Over time, your thoughts have become less muddled and you only hear the voices once a week or so, usually when you are alone. Today, you are being discharged from hospital, and you attended a long meeting to help decide the arrangements for your care outside hospital. Unfortunately, you did not entirely agree with what was said and you have asked to speak with the doctor to clarify some important questions.

You want to know whether you will have any contact with the psychiatrists or nurses.

You would like to go back to work, and want to know when you can.

You want to know when you can stop taking the injection

45. Compliance

You are a forty-five-year-old man, who has suffered from schizophrenia for the last ten years. You have been admitted to hospital four times over these years. All of your admissions to hospital have occurred because you have stopped taking your medication, because you don't think you are mentally ill. On each occasion, your illness has subsequently become worse, and you have responded to your paranoia and the voices you hear in your head, by attacking neighbours or strangers in the street. You have had to be detained against your will in hospital for up to several months. This has caused great disruption in your life. You have stopped working in your job as an accountant, and your family now survives on your wife's income. You have lost all your friends, and have no motivation to keep active. You spend most of your time at home, watching television, or reading books. Although you don't think that you need medication, you can see some of the beneficial effects medication has had on your life, such as keeping you out of hospital, allowing you to get on with your family, and most important of all, making the voices you hear on a daily basis, less intrusive and distressing.

This is the last day of your fifth admission to hospital. This doctor wants to talk to you about your medication and why you need to take it. You would like to know what you can do to help you remember to take your medication. Please follow any instructions that the doctor gives you.

30. Discussion with senior colleague

Introduces self.
Asks for advice.
Confirms it is appropriate to discuss a difficult case at this time.

Introduction   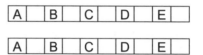

Appropriateness of call | A | | B | | C | | D | | E | |

⌘ Describes the basic demographics of the patient.

⌘ Also includes mention of current legal status and duration of inpatient stay.

⌘ Confirms current diagnosis and treatment plan from medical notes.

⌘ Gives an account of events leading up to the assessment of the patient.

Basic patient details | A | | B | | C | | D | | E | |

Describes scenario | A | | B | | C | | D | | E | |

⌘ Elaborates on details of his assessment:

- presentation
- circumstances of admission
- current mental state including mood, delusions, and suicidal thoughts or plans
- highlights patients feelings of guilt, hopelessness and worthlessness.

⌘ Specifies patient's current level of insight into his condition and need for help.

⌘ Confirms patient's intention to leave hospital and/or attempt(s) to leave already made.

Current mental state | A | | B | | C | | D | | E | |

Highlights suicidal thoughts or plans   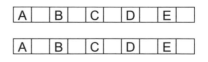

❄ Asks about criteria for detention under the Mental Health Act, or states them at onset— risk to patient's own health, safety or for the protection of others.

❄ Suggests that detention may be appropriate.

❄ Asks for advice on the issue of further detention.

Detention criteria   [A| |B| |C| |D| |E|]

Factual knowledge   [A| |B| |C| |D| |E|]

Ending   [A| |B| |C| |D| |E|]

Global rating   [A| |B| |C| |D| |E|]

31. Explanation of diagnosis: borderline personality disorder

It is usual to preface any discussion with relatives by stating that you would have asked the patient herself for permission to talk to her stepmother about her diagnosis and management plans.

Introduces self.
Is sensitive and empathic.
Listens and uses appropriate language.

Introduction   [A| |B| |C| |D| |E|]

❄ Discusses the current admission:

- reasons for the admission
- any concerns she has about discharge from hospital.

❄ Addresses the main issue of diagnosis:

❖ Explain that the diagnosis is correctly labelled 'emotionally unstable personality disorder, of the emotional type'
❖ Explain that it comprises 'an enduring pattern of behaviour that reflects difficulties in her personality development'.
❖ These difficulties are pervasive in nature, that is, they have an impact on several domains in her life such as her behaviour, emotions, thinking and response to stress from early adulthood onwards. Her personality problems cause distress to herself, others and society as a whole. At a personal level, they cause difficulties in interpersonal relationships, and her occupational and social life.

The key point at this stage is to mention that the difficulties in her personality are not attributable to mental illness, drug misuse or physical illnesses.

General introduction:

Borderline personality disorder is a complex condition and presents differently in different individuals. Perhaps we should start by talking about what is known about the disorder in general and then talk about your daughter in more detail.

It is said to affect about 2% of the general population. It is a disorder in which the individual has problems in maintaining relationships or have a pattern of unstable relationships. They find it hard to know themselves and do not have a stable sense of themselves. They feel empty a lot of the time and are unable express their true feelings at times. They are impulsive and this is reflected in their behaviour, be it misusing drugs and alcohol, or engaging in several brief, intense relationships. They fear abandonment and will go to great lengths to prevent this from happening, such as taking overdoses to prevent a partner from leaving.

General introduction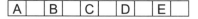

⌘ Offer more details of common symptoms and signs:

It is also known that people with BPD, swing between idealizing and devaluing people in relationships, which in turn could lead to them classifying people in their mind as being either all good or all bad. We call this 'splitting' people into two groups, and it can occur even within the setting of the ward, when some staff are labelled as 'caring' and others as the exact opposite. The side to which one is classified can change from day to day. Because we know this occurs, we try to present a united front to such patients, so that the messages they get are exactly the same from all involved in their care.

Patients with borderline disorder harm themselves by taking overdoses of prescribed and non-prescribed medication. They also make suicidal gestures or attempts. They suffer from mood swings, anger outbursts and anxiety symptoms. In stressful situations some patients hear voices and feel suspicious about others, what we label as 'transient psychotic experiences', and they may need treatment for these episodes.

Patients are aware of the pain and distress they cause by their actions to themselves and others, but feel unable to control fully their behaviour. They may also feel victimised, blamed, and criticised by others, including carers. From your part, you may feel misunderstood and constantly let down by their behaviour.

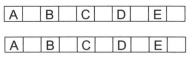

Sensitive, non-judgmental approach

Simple language

Factual knowledge | A | B | C | D | E |

⌘ Discusses possible management options.

> *Treatment for the symptoms experienced usually consists of medication and talking therapy. Anti-depressants help to minimize depressed moods and reduce impulsivity. Mood stabilizers may help with mood swings and irritability. Occasionally, anti-psychotics are given to help with psychotic experiences such as hearing voices, and also to help with impulse control.*
>
> *The psychological or talking therapies include long-term psychodynamic psychotherapy, that explores the development of behaviours in the context of the patient's early development and way of interacting with others. There are also shorter term treatments such as dialectical behavioral therapy (DBT) and cognitive behavioral therapy (CBT) which are more focused on looking at faulty ways of thinking and dealing with emotions.*

⌘ Addresses any questions that she may have.

Empathic | A | B | C | D | E |

Adequate explanation | A | B | C | D | E |

Addresses concerns | A | B | C | D | E |

Ending | A | B | C | D | E |

Global rating | A | B | C | D | E |

32. Explanation of side-effects: antipsychotics

Introduces self.
Explains purpose of discussion.

Introduction | A | B | C | D | E |

Sets agenda | A | B | C | D | E |

⌘ Clarifies current medication:

- name, dose, when started
- reasons why she was started on it
- ask what she already knows of the medication.

⌘ Has she had any positive effects so far?

⌘ Has she had any side-effects?

  • if so, what? When did it begin?

⌘ Addresses concerns.

⌘ Reassures patient.

Current situation |A| |B| |C| |D| |E| |

Positive effects |A| |B| |C| |D| |E| |

Rapport |A| |B| |C| |D| |E| |

Sensitivity |A| |B| |C| |D| |E| |

⌘ Explains, in simple language, the mechanism of action, precautions, and side-effects of the drug she is currently on.

  • two main groups of drugs used to treat psychotic symptoms, namely the typical and atypical antipsychotic medications
  • briefly explain the role of chemical messengers in the brain such as dopamine and serotonin.
  • explain the risk of treatment emergent side-effects on these drugs due to their wide variety of action on different parts of the brain.

⌘ Enquire about any specific side-effects she may be concerned about:

  • concerns regarding pregnancy.
  • concerns about menstrual irregularities
  • concerns about her sexual drive
  • concerns about breast enlargement or discharge.

⌘ Clarify if any of these side-effects emerged after starting the medication.

⌘ Explore any other side-effects, and when they occurred. Are they in any way related to the dose of medication prescribed?

Explanation of mode of action |A| |B| |C| |D| |E| |

Elicits concerns |A| |B| |C| |D| |E| |

⌘ Explain about the side-effects systematically, starting from brain, heart, digestive system, bones, hormonal and endocrine systems, and effects on weight.

The list of side-effects varies with each drug. You will need to familiarise yourself with the common ones for each of the commonly prescribed drugs. Remember that although there are less of the old side-effects with atypicals, there are also a whole host of new ones. For example, you would need to discuss weight gain and altered glucose metabolism when talking about olanzapine.

⌘ Explain about the need for frequent monitoring of various parameters when on these drugs. There are, of course, some general tests including liver functions tests and urea and electrolytes, along with other physical investigations such as an ECG for most patients about to commence on antipsychotics. There are also drug specific tests. For example, it is important to mention serum prolactin levels for risperidone, and fasting blood glucose for olanzapine, both before and after starting the drugs.

⌘ Offer to give patient information leaflets on the drug.

⌘ Address any questions that she may have.

⌘ Offer to discuss this further, and state that she can opt for an alternative drug should she wish.

Explanation of general side-effects	A	B	C	D	E
Explanation of specific side-effects	A	B	C	D	E
Factual knowledge	A	B	C	D	E
Ending	A	B	C	D	E
Global rating	A	B	C	D	E

33. Management of weight gain

Introduces self
Explains purpose of discussion

Introduction	A	B	C	D	E
Sets agenda	A	B	C	D	E

⌘ Explores:

- current weight and height. If possible, to calculate BMI.
- weight before commencing medication
- pattern of weight gain — was it more evident earlier on? Has the weight gain slowed down or stopped?
- has the weight gain changed with the dose of medication?
- does he believe the weight gain is solely due to the medication?
- has he experienced any other side-effects?

⌘ Explores adverse effects of current situation:

- has he noticed any problems with the additional weight?
- does he know what his ideal weight should be?
- is he aware of any of the risks of being overweight, such as the increased risk of developing diabetes and heart disease?

Explores current state | A | | B | | C | | D | | E | |

⌘ Explains the risk of weight gain on antipsychotics:

- that it is a known complication, though it is said that the overall gain occurs in the first few months, and plateaus thereafter
- does he recall being warned about this side effect before it was started?

⌘ Explains the need for weight control measures to be instituted at the time medication was started.

Explanation | A | | B | | C | | D | | E | |

⌘ Explores lifestyle factors and their contribution to his weight/current situation:

- eating habits
- exercise
- alcohol
- smoking.

⌘ Explores attempts to lose weight:

- avoidance of fatty foods
- diets
- use of any medication.

⌘ Attempts to get help:

- GP
- dietician
- well man clinic
- advice from CPN or others.

Elicits lifestyle factors | A | | B | | C | | D | | E | |

Explains effects on weight | A | | B | | C | | D | | E | |

Attempts to get help and lose weight | A | | B | | C | | D | | E | |

⌘ Offers help:

- through GP and dietician
- through CPN support
- if available, refer to a weight management clinic
- further discussion about related topics such as healthy eating, and lifestyle changes.

Sensitive | A | B | C | D | E |

Offers help | A | B | C | D | E |

⌘ Further explores any other problems with current medication:

- offer to try a dose reduction
- offer close weight monitoring in clinic, and monitoring of lipid profile, through regular blood tests.

⌘ Discusses the option of changing medication:

- possible side-effects of alternative medication
- gives patient information leaflets for patient to read through
- addresses any questions that patient may have.

⌘ Discusses whether the patient is willing to continue on current medication.

Considers alternatives | A | B | C | D | E |

Addresses patient's concerns | A | B | C | D | E |

Ending | A | B | C | D | E |

Global rating | A | B | C | D | E |

34. Explanation of action: antipsychotics

Introduces self.
Explains purpose of discussion.

Introduction | A | B | C | D | E |

Sets agenda | A | B | C | D | E |

⌘ Clarifies current medication:

- name, dose, when started
- reasons why she was started on it
- ask what she already knows of the medication

- has she had any positive effects so far?
- has she had any side effects? If so, what? When did it begin?

⌘ Addresses concerns.

⌘ Reassures patient.

Current situation ||A| |B| |C| |D| |E| ||

Positive effects ||A| |B| |C| |D| |E| ||

Rapport ||A| |B| |C| |D| |E| ||

Sensitive ||A| |B| |C| |D| |E| ||

⌘ Explains in simple language the mechanism of action:

❖ Briefly explains the role of chemical messengers in the brain such as dopamine and serotonin, and how it is thought that psychotic symptoms, such as hearing hallucinatory voices and experiencing paranoid thoughts, are thought to occur as a result of an imbalance of these messengers.
❖ Explains that the main drugs used to treat schizophrenia act on the levels of the different messengers to bring them back to normal.
❖ Gives an equivalent scenario from physical medicine, such as diabetics needing to have their insulin levels restored to allow for proper functioning.

> *Schizophrenia is a syndrome, or collection of symptoms and signs that is believed to be due to a chemical imbalance in the brain. Research evidence suggests that there is an imbalance in the concentration of certain chemicals in the nerve cells of the brain. The two important ones are called dopamine and serotonin. It is believed that when the concentration of dopamine in the brain cells is excessive, they do not function normally, and this in turn makes us feel different and experience unusual thoughts and perceptions. For example, some people hear voices when there's no one around, or experience paranoia. The medication you are taking is called an antipsychotic, because it acts to alter the levels of these chemicals in your brain, and thereby stop your experiences or at least make them more bearable.*

⌘ Explains in some detail about the various mediation options

- two main groups of drugs used to treat psychotic symptoms; namely, the typical and atypical antipsychotic medications
- atypicals are nowadays recommended by the Government to be used as first line treatments for schizophrenia.

⌘ Explain the risk of treatment emergent side-effects on these drugs due to their wide variety of action on different parts of the brain.

⌘ Explores her concerns about weight gain and ways in which this might be managed (see question 33 in this book).

Simple terms used

A | B | C | D | E

Factual knowledge

A | B | C | D | E

⌘ Explains about the need to continue medication for symptom remission:

- nowadays it is advised that patients continue on antipsychotic medication to keep symptoms under control.
- this will also entail psychiatric or GP follow-up and may also need regular blood tests to monitor for some side effects.
- explore the ongoing benefits of continuing medication
- offer patient information leaflets.

⌘ Enquires about whether the patient intends to continue with her medication:

- offer alternatives to current medication, including reduction of dose.

⌘ Explains about possible side effects of any new medication.

Benefits of continuing medication

A | B | C | D | E

Alternatives

A | B | C | D | E

Ending

A | B | C | D | E

Global rating

A | B | C | D | E

35. Explanation of cognitive therapy for depression

Introduces self.
Establishes rapport.

Introduction

A | B | C | D | E

⌘ Elicits brief history:

- duration of symptoms, and severity
- treatments tried, and their effectiveness
- what has prompted this interview?
- what does she already know about cognitive therapy?

It appears that your illness has not responded to three antidepressants and you continue to have negative thoughts about yourself and the world. Perhaps we can now look at what you wanted to discuss. Could you tell me what you already know about cognitive therapy?

Brief history

A	B	C	D	E

Elicits prior knowledge

A	B	C	D	E

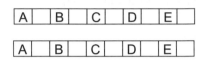

❀ Brief explanation of what psychotherapy in general and cognitive therapy specifically entail:

Cognitive therapy is one of the talking therapies or psychological therapies which involves listening and talking with a therapist. It is usually offered along with antidepressant medication. In cognitive therapy, it is thought that understanding your thinking can influence how you feel and behave. So, if your thinking is altered, such as always thinking negatively about yourself, the therapist will work with you to explore why you believe that is true. Once you can see that way of thinking is flawed, you can then look at other ways of thinking, which are more helpful and might influence your mood in a positive way. Cognitive therapy is different from some of the other psychotherapies, because it is time-limited, with a fixed number of sessions, and looks at present day difficulties, rather than those in the past. You will be given work to do at home before sessions. The homework involves recording thoughts and beliefs, and after later sessions, looks at how you test your own incorrect assumptions or beliefs.

❀ Explanation about negative cognitive triad:

- negative views of self, world and the future
- the process of reactivation of negative cognitions when exposed to a critical incident.

❀ Explanation of cognitive distortions or 'thinking errors':

- all-or-nothing thinking, over-generalisation, magnification, selective abstraction, arbitrary inference, and labelling

❀ Explains how they lead people to look selectively at information that conforms to how they see things, and to discard information that does not conform.

General description

A	B	C	D	E

Negative cognitive triad

A	B	C	D	E

Thinking errors

A	B	C	D	E

⌘ More detailed explanation | A | B | C | D | E |

The therapist will play a very active part in your treatment, and will focus the sessions onto achieving specific tasks. There are usually ten to twenty sessions in total. The therapist will help you to identify your problematic thoughts and beliefs, and will then help to find solutions. You will need to maintain a diary to keep a record of your negative thoughts and thinking errors. The therapist will work with you and help you to challenge them and look at alternative explanations or possibilities. Eventually you will learn to replace them with more positive thoughts.

The whole idea of this therapy is to help you to see how you have been unreasonably critical about yourself, your future and the world in general, and to modify your current thinking. In essence, the logical basis of negative thoughts is challenged and you are helped to identify positive thoughts.

In later stages, you will perform 'experiments' to test negative underlying assumptions about yourself, which we call 'schemas', and put to use the newly learnt positive thoughts and coping skills.

Explanation | A | B | C | D | E |

Factual knowledge | A | B | C | D | E |

Addresses patient's enquiries and concerns | A | B | C | D | E |

Ending | A | B | C | D | E |

Global rating | A | B | C | D | E |

36. Explanation of diagnosis: schizophrenia

Introduces self.
Is sensitive and empathic.
Listens and uses appropriate language.

Introduction | A | B | C | D | E |

⌘ Discusses the current admission:

- reasons for the admission
- any concerns he has about discharge from hospital
- address the main issue of diagnosis.

⌘ Explain that his illness is called 'schizophrenia.'

✥ Enquires about what he already knows about schizophrenia.

General introduction to the illness:

Schizophrenia is a disorder of the brain. It affects around one in a hundred people and is seen throughout the world. It is thought to be due to abnormalities in the nerve cells of the brain. We are not completely certain about the cause of this illness. Some of it may be hereditary, and the rest may be due to environmental effects. It is thought that in some individuals who have a genetic vulnerability, some sort of stress or even the use of certain illicit drugs can trigger the onset of the illness.

The term 'schizophrenia' itself describes a split personality, but although that is how it may be perceived by the public, that's not what is actually happening.

It is a condition in which the individual has disordered thinking and perception, which in turn could affect their ability to understand normal events happening around them. The illness manifests itself as 'psychosis', which is a term used to describe some of the key features of the illness. For example, hearing hallucinatory voices (when there is no one about) is one type of psychotic experience. Many patients also have unusual, fixed beliefs, which we call 'delusions.' Examples include believing that they are being persecuted, or that there is a conspiracy to harm them in some way. The third symptom that can be termed 'psychotic' is the experience of having disorganised thinking, which can result in the patient appearing to talk nonsense or not being understood at all.

Usually, a diagnosis of schizophrenia is made only after finding out about the person's behaviour (from themselves or their carers and by interview and observation) and after they have been experiencing the psychotic symptoms for at least one month. Some patients suffer for months or longer without their family or friends knowing.

The course of schizophrenia varies from one patient to the next. All we know is that about 15% of those who have a psychotic breakdown make a complete recovery. The remaining 85% have a fluctuating course of symptoms, with relapses and recovery periods for the rest of their lives. They may go on to develop the long term 'negative' symptoms of schizophrenia, such as apathy, lack of motivation, poor communication skills, and impaired social interaction. Unfortunately, we can't tell in advance which group a person will fall into. However, we do have several different treatment options to try to bring symptoms under control, and to allow patients to get back to their lives. The treatment that is available includes medication and talking therapies

Concise introduction	A	B	C	D	E

Simple language	A	B	C	D	E

Factual knowledge	A	B	C	D	E

⌘ Address any questions or concerns the patient may have.

With regard to going back to work, it is advisable that this is done in a gradual manner, as stress of any kind is linked to a worsening of symptoms. The first step is to make a decision to inform employers and then decide how to proceed. Usually, employers are supportive, and one can look at going back to work part time initially, before building up to full time commitment. Alternatively, one can look at alternatives to returning to the old job, by exploring skills and training that can be used in a different or related job.

⌘ Attempt to illustrate aspects of diagnosis with relation to patient's symptoms

Try to expand on some of the patient's symptoms to show how they would be considered to represent mental illness. It is important to use the correct phrases, as you have to avoid appearing judgmental or confrontational. And, remember that what we as clinicians perceive as psychosis, is perceived as very real by the patient. In the scenario, as it appears, the patient had recovered from acute illness, you might phrase questions starting with:

> *Do you remember when you first came here, you were convinced that you were being followed by MI5. This may have been considered as a delusion of persecution. You could also hear peoples' voices coming from the walls. We think that this meant that you were experiencing hallucinatory voices. At the time, I'm sure these felt very real to you.*

⌘ Offer to give patient information leaflets about schizophrenia:

- also, say that you can give him numbers for various national support agencies like Rethink (formerly known as the National Schizophrenia Fellowship), MIND, and Saneline, who can support both him and his family.
- offer to put him in touch with the local advocacy service for patients
- suggest that the option of a second opinion on the diagnosis is always available.

⌘ Expand on the importance of medication:

> *The risk of relapse in those who discontinue medication is high, and current recommendations are that antipsychotic medication should be continued for up to one to two years after a relapse* (NICE, 2002). *Also, it is advised that following supervised, gradual withdrawal from antipsychotic medication, monitoring for signs and symptoms of relapse should go on for at least two years after the most recent acute episode.*

Addresses patient's concerns about work

| A | B | C | D | E |

Explores symptoms in relation to diagnosis

| A | B | C | D | E |

Sources of support and information | A | | B | | C | | D | | E | |

Importance of medication | A | | B | | C | | D | | E | |

Ending | A | | B | | C | | D | | E | |

Global rating | A | | B | | C | | D | | E | |

37. Breaking bad news

Initial steps before approaching the patient (said to the examiner):

❖ Check the information is correct — what was the cause of death?
❖ Briefly review patient's notes to learn about diagnosis, and current management plan. Has there been any discussion about the potential bereavement with staff on either ward? Was he aware of the seriousness of her illness? Did he discuss his wife's condition with the medical staff? Does he have any other source of support? Find out if his key nurse would like to be with you when you speak to him. Is it thought that he may have been anticipating his wife's death?
❖ Speak with staff to see whether he can see his wife's body. Are any other preparations being made, such as a post-mortem examination?
❖ Check whether other relatives have been informed.
❖ Ask to see him in a private, quiet room.

Preparatory steps | A | | B | | C | | D | | E | |

⌘ Introduces self and other staff member present.

Introduction | A | | B | | C | | D | | E | |

⌘ Begins with a direct statement:

> *I am afraid I have some bad news for you. I have been told by the staff at the dialysis unit that your wife has just passed away. I am sorry to have to bring you this news at this time.*

⌘ Waits for patient's response:

This is not an interview scenario, and so you will have to be guided by the patient's response to the news you have given him.

If patient wants to know more, explain what you know, using clear and simple terms. State that you have spoken with staff on the unit, and that he can, if he wishes, speak directly with them:

- offer to return later if he wishes
- ask whether he needs anything at the moment.

Sensitivity | A | B | C | D | E |

Use of language | A | B | C | D | E |

⌘ Gently explores patient's reaction to the news:

- was he expecting this to happen?
- when did he last see her? How had she been at that time?
- was he aware of how ill she had been and spoken to the doctors?

⌘ Allows patient time to ventilate his feelings:

- he may go through the initial stages of grief, starting with a period of numbness. This may progress to distress and anxiety. You will have to deal with the emotions as they become evident. The key point is to listen, and be supportive. Offer information if you have it.

Explores patient reaction | A | B | C | D | E |

Allows ventilation of emotions | A | B | C | D | E |

Provides information | A | B | C | D | E |

⌘ Explores how patient wants to proceed

- Would he like to speak to the staff about going to see his wife?
- Would he prefer for staff from this ward to speak to staff at the renal unit to find out what will happen next?
- What would he like to do next?

Further practical steps | A | B | C | D | E |

⌘ Offers support from staff:

- acknowledge this is a difficult time and state that staff members are on hand at all times should he need to speak to anyone
- also offers practical help from staff
- mention that when patients die in hospital, postmortems may be conducted if there are any questions that are unexplained, and that if this is the case, the staff on the renal unit would let him know. They would also want to discuss any funeral arrangements directly with him.

Offers support | A | B | C | D | E |

Ending | A | B | C | D | E |

Global rating | A | B | C | D | E |

38. Discontinuation of lithium

Introduces self.
Confirms reason for discussion.
Establishes rapport.

Introduction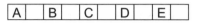

⌘ Elicits salient features of history:

- diagnosis
- duration of symptoms
- current medication and dose
- current mental state. Is she depressed or elated?
- has she been under any stress recently? What sort of support does she have at home?
- has she had any specific side effects? Ask about tremor, distaste in tongue, polyuria, constipation, weight gain and other thyroid related symptoms.

History | A | | B | | C | | D | | E | |
|---|---|---|---|---|---|---|---|---|---|

Current side-effects | A | | B | | C | | D | | E | |
|---|---|---|---|---|---|---|---|---|---|

⌘ Elicits patient's knowledge about lithium and it's role as a mood stabiliser:

- what has being on lithium meant for her? Has it been of any benefit?
- has it had any effect on her illness?
- does she attribute her long history of being well to the drug?
- has she tried to come off it before? Was it a sudden discontinuation or gradual reduction under supervision? What was the result?
- is she aware of potential side effects?
- has she had regular blood tests? Does she know why she has been having them?
- what are her main concerns at the moment?
- side-effects
- duration of treatment
- Availability of alternatives.

⌘ Explanation of mechanism of action:

> *Lithium is a mood stabiliser, which has been shown to be effective in the treatment of mania and in prevention of relapse in bipolar disorder or 'manic depression'. The exact mechanism of action is not known, though it is thought that the drug stabilises the outer membranes of nerve cells in the brain. This is turn helps to stabilise the extremes of mood experienced by patients.*
>
> *The drug itself has been in use for around forty years, and many patients have been on continuous treatment with it for several years.*

⌘ Expands on side-effects:

> *There are several side-effects, some of which are mild, and others which can be potentially life-threatening. The milder side-effects include stomach upset, weight gain, fine tremor, fatigue and drowsiness, excessive thirst, passing water frequently, dry mouth, metallic taste, and acne. The more serious side-effects include damage to the kidneys and the thyroid gland, which are more long-term effects and are monitored for by having regular three-monthly blood tests. There is also said to be a risk of cognitive and memory impairment. In addition, if the level of lithium in the blood goes too high, it can be toxic to the brain, causing seizures, coma and even death. Again, this is carefully monitored by ensuring that the levels in the blood keep within a safe range.*

She may already know that blood levels can be affected by diarrhoea, vomiting, impaired kidney functioning and drug interactions, and that these are also conditions for which she has to see her GP for urgent advice.

Elicits current knowledge | A | | B | | C | | D | | E | |

Addresses patient's concerns | A | | B | | C | | D | | E | |

Explains action, side-effects and precautions | A | | B | | C | | D | | E | |

Simple language | A | | B | | C | | D | | E | |

Factual knowledge | A | | B | | C | | D | | E | |

⌘ Explain the risk of refractoriness to lithium treatment once it is discontinued, as well as the increased risk of relapse of illness with abrupt withdrawal.

⌘ Explores her knowledge about alternatives to lithium:

- unlicensed drugs, which are normally used as antiepileptics, include carbamazepine, and sodium valproate.
- valproic acid is a newly licensed drug that can be used in patients unresponsive to lithium.

⌘ Addresses any questions she may have.

⌘ Elicits whether her views have changed.

⌘ Offers patient information leaflets and a further appointment to discuss options.

Discusses alternatives | A | | B | | C | | D | | E | |

Ending | A | | B | | C | | D | | E | |

Global rating | A | | B | | C | | D | | E | |

For further information see Baldessarini *et al*, 1996; Bauer, 1994.

39. Explanation of vascular dementia

Introduces self.
Establishes rapport.
Shows empathy.
Checks existing knowledge.
Inquires to what extend the information applies to her husband.

Introduction | A | | B | | C | | D | | E | |

⌘ Asks about her own experiences:

- current situation
- duration of symptoms
- progress
- level of functioning
- specific difficulties.

Elicits history | A | | B | | C | | D | | E | |

⌘ Enquires about risk-factors:

- hypertension
- smoking
- diabetes
- high cholesterol
- heart disease.

Explores risk factors | A | | B | | C | | D | | E | |

⌘ Explains what vascular dementia is:

- an illness of the brain, which leads to confusion, memory-problems and disorientation
- it can also cause difficulties in other areas of functioning, such as self-care, language, practical skills, personality and mood
- it occurs mainly in the elderly, and is a chronic condition, which only deteriorates over time.
- the deterioration often occurs in a stepwise fashion, with plateaus for short durations of time followed by abrupt falls in functioning.

Basic description of illness | A | | B | | C | | D | | E | |

⌘ Gives information about causes:

- it is caused by infarcts, or areas of brain-damage due to an obstruction in the blood-supply to parts of the brain
- there can be several infarcts, which may vary in size, and affect different parts of the brain
- The infarct may present as a stroke (cerebrovascular attack [CVA]) or a mini-stroke (transient ischaemic attack [TIA]) or it may even go unnoticed
- there may be other signs of vascular disease like a heart-attack
- factors like high blood pressure, diabetes, smoking, and high blood lipids also contribute to the risk of developing the dementia.

Discussion of aetiology | A | | B | | C | | D | | E | |

⌘ Explains differences from Alzheimer's dementia:

- the causes for Alzheimer's dementia are less clear
- progress in Alzheimer's disease is more gradual
- Alzheimer's disease affects the brain more globally
- in Alzheimer's you tend to see a more widespread deterioration
- in vascular dementia certain areas of functioning can be affected, while others can remain intact
- in vascular dementia people tend to be aware of the deterioration in their condition until much later in the illness
- depression is more common in vascular dementia.

Contrast with Alzheimer's dementia | A | | B | | C | | D | | E | |

⌘ Discusses prognosis:

- mentions that the condition of patients tends to deteriorate in a stepwise fashion. The rate of this can vary. Patients can be stable for a long time, before they have a further deterioration. Over time they become increasingly dependent and towards the end of the illness, may well need high levels of care.

Prognosis | A | | B | | C | | D | | E | |

⌘ Explains that modifying risk factors may slow down the progression:

- good regulation of diabetes
- healthy diet and weight loss
- giving up smoking
- anti-coagulants, eg. aspirin.

Modifying risk factors | A | | B | | C | | D | | E | |

❈ Suggests other possibilities for support:

- home care
- day care
- CPN and social work support
- carer support groups
- voluntary organisations
- Alzheimer's society
- respite care
- residential or nursing-home care
- other types of medication like calming drugs or antidepressants.

It is important to inform her that the new anti-dementia drugs she may have heard of, are in fact for people with Alzheimer's dementia rather than vascular dementia.

Discuss support available |A| |B| |C| |D| |E| |

Addresses patient's questions or concerns |A| |B| |C| |D| |E| |

Ending |A| |B| |C| |D| |E| |

Global rating |A| |B| |C| |D| |E| |

40. Explanation of psychodynamic psychotherapy

Introduces self.
Establishes rapport.
Clarifies reasons for the consultation.
Enquires about her own knowledge of the subject.
Asks whether she knows anyone who had psychotherapy.
Asks about expectations and concerns.

Communication |A| |B| |C| |D| |E| |

Question-framing |A| |B| |C| |D| |E| |

Basic aspects of psychotherapy:

- ❖ Psychotherapy is an active therapeutic process of listening and talking.
- ❖ The therapist encourages you to talk freely about your experiences.
- ❖ You will look at your thoughts, feelings and actions in specific situations.
- ❖ It is important to talk openly, even if things are painful or don't make sense.
- ❖ In this way, you will try to discover common themes in your current difficulties.
- ❖ By understanding your problems better you may find it easier to deal with them.

Basic principles |A| |B| |C| |D| |E| |

Information about the therapist:

❖ The psychotherapist may have a medical background, or may have a related background such as social work or nursing.
❖ The therapist is impartial and has to maintain confidentiality.
❖ The therapist usually discusses your case regularly with a supervisor throughout the time you have therapy. Discussing matters with the supervisor helps your therapist to get an external view of how therapy is progressing.

Therapist details |A| |B| |C| |D| |E| |

Explanation of some of the underlying themes of therapy:

❖ Your relationship with the therapist may mirror previous relationships you have had and help you to understand how you respond to other people.
❖ Some of your interaction may reflect the way you responded to your parents as a child.

Transference |A| |B| |C| |D| |E| |

❖ It may not always be an easy process.
❖ You may feel that you are not getting anywhere, or sometimes that your problems are getting worse.
❖ We all have feelings, thoughts and experiences we are not aware of or want to ignore. It may be hard to look at some areas, because it's too painful.
❖ The therapist may try to help you with these areas by suggesting possible explanations and will encourage you to look at past events.

Resistance |A| |B| |C| |D| |E| |

Therapeutic setting

❖ Consistency and structure for each session are important.
❖ Meetings with the therapist will be on a regular basis, usually once a week.
❖ Sessions can also be more frequent, eg. twice a week.
❖ In most cases a session will last for about fifty minutes. It is expected that you will be on time for sessions. In turn, the therapist will try to see you at the same time and place each week
❖ The length of the therapy varies from about three months to a year or more.

Therapy boundaries |A| |B| |C| |D| |E| |

Outcome:

❖ Towards the end of the therapy you will hopefully have a better understanding of your difficulties, and will be more confident in dealing with them.
❖ The positive effects include reduction in personal distress, and improvement in your relationships and self-esteem.

Expected outcomes   A B C D E

Ending   A B C D E

Global rating   A B C D E

41. Referral of a confused patient to a medical colleague

Introduces self.
Is professional and patient.
Gives a clear and concise history.
Explains arguments for referral clearly.

Communication   A B C D E

Professional manner   A B C D E

⌘ Gives history of circumstances on admission:

- personal details
- initial presentation
- previous medical history
- reasons for admission to psychiatric ward.

Presentation on admission   A B C D E

⌘ Explains reasons for suspected delirium:

- acute onset
- absence of previous psychiatric history
- lack of evidence for dementia
- fluctuation in level of consciousness
- disorientation
- incoherent speech
- presence of visual hallucinations
- disrupted sleep wake cycle.

Symptoms of delirium   A B C D E

⌘ Mentions possible causes for delirium:

- raised temperature
- urinary tract infection
- other infections
- electrolyte imbalance
- propanolol
- vascular (TIA/CVA)
- other causes
- combination of any of the above.

Elaborates possible causes of delirium |A| |B| |C| |D| |E| |

⌘ Explains reasons for referral:

- need for further medical assessment to exclude serious underlying problems
- possible need for further investigations
- limited capability for medical management on psychiatric ward.

Reasons for referral |A| |B| |C| |D| |E| |

⌘ Offers further advice and consultation if necessary:

- makes suggestions for management of delirium
- expresses willingness to take back the patient for assessment and treatment of any underlying mental illness after medical treatment has stabilised her condition.

Ending |A| |B| |C| |D| |E| |

Global rating |A| |B| |C| |D| |E| |

42. Agoraphobia and behavioural therapy

Establishes rapport.
Is polite and empathic.
Does not use jargon.
Is sensitive to patient's concerns.

Listening skills |A| |B| |C| |D| |E| |

Verbal facilitation |A| |B| |C| |D| |E| |

Use of language |A| |B| |C| |D| |E| |

⌘ Explores the extent and severity of her symptoms:

- onset, duration and progression of anxiety symptoms
- are they generalised, or restricted to certain situations?
- associated psychological and physical symptoms of low grade anxiety
- ask for restlessness, poor concentration, irritability, occasional dry mouth, rapid breathing, tiredness, muscle aches
- ask about panic attacks
- situation, duration, and specific physical and psychological symptoms
- catastrophic thoughts such as that she is dying, or having a heart attack:

What was going through your mind at the time?

- as about breathlessness, palpitations ('as if your heart was racing'), sweating, dry mouth, nausea, vomiting, chest pains, paleness, dizziness, tremor, blurred vision, paraesthesia ('tingling in the fingers and toes').

Explores anxiety symptoms

Assesses associated
physical/psychological symptoms

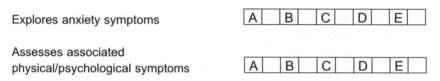

æ Explores the extent of avoidance and specific avoidant behaviours:

What sorts of things do you do to avoid becoming anxious?

- how difficult are these behaviours/actions? Do they make her feel less anxious? How often does she have to do them? How much time is spent in the average day avoiding her anxiety? Ask for more examples.
- are there times when she does not notice her anxiety, for just short periods of time? How does she feel at these times?
- ask about anticipatory anxiety — does it restrict her life in any way? Does it prevent her from doing things she normally enjoys?

Explores avoidance | A | B | C | D | E |

æ Introduces behavioural therapy as a possible mode of therapy:

From what you have said so far, I think that I now have a fair idea of the extent to which your anxiety affects your everyday life. I also have clearer picture of the various things you do to avoid your anxiety. Let's now talk about how we might be able to help you with your problem. Your GP referred you here to see if behavioural therapy might help. Have you heard of it before?

Behavioural therapy is one of the non-medication treatments, which involves doing less anxiety-provoking tasks or behaviours, initially in the mind and then later in reality, in a structured and hierarchical way, so as to overcome a larger anxiety-provoking problem. It is usually done over a fixed number of sessions. The main idea behind it is that our everyday behaviour is the result of what we think and how we feel. So if we can alter our behaviour in a small way, it may lead to a change in the way we think and feel about a particular task.

For example, if there is a large task ahead of us, like going to work on a daily basis, it may initially seem impossible to do. We might even be doing other things to try and avoid or reduce the anxiety around the main task. In behaviour therapy, we would look at the main task in detail, and decide on how to break it up into smaller, more achievable tasks. For example, you could start by imagining going out for just a few minutes to do essential shopping. The next step might be to actually do exactly that. Then you might work your way up to going out for a meal for just an hour, and so on. You would need to decide on exactly what to do for each task, and then rank them in order of difficulty. The 'avoidant behaviours' would also be looked at and we would explore ways of stopping them completely. You would then systematically work your way through the smaller, but increasingly more difficult tasks and eventually, you should be able to perform the large, difficult task with only minimal anxiety. The whole process may be combined with a talking therapy like cognitive therapy. If we wanted to do combined 'cognitive behavioural therapy', then we would start at the beginning and also look at our feelings and thought processes in relation to the main task. As the therapy progresses, we would then look at other ways of thinking, which do not lead to our anxious feelings, and over time replace the old, negative ways of thinking with newer, more constructive and more positive ways of thinking. Eventually, we hope that when faced with a similar problem in the future, the positive way you think about it, will affect how you feel and in consequence how you react to, or behave, in the situation.

⌘ Offers to give her a leaflet that would explain the therapy in more detail. Also, state that she can have more time to think about it. Ask whether she has any questions.

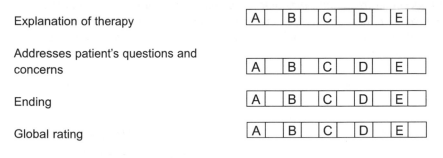

Explanation of therapy   A B C D E

Addresses patient's questions and concerns   A B C D E

Ending   A B C D E

Global rating   A B C D E

43. Lithium in pregnancy

There are two key points in this OSCE. Firstly, how you convey this potentially upsetting news to the patient. Secondly, how you present the relevant information in a balanced manner so as to allow the patient to make an informed choice. You will also need to end by recording the decision, and conveying it to relevant colleagues.

Introduces self.
Asks about reason for the urgent appointment.
Reassures the patient that she has acted appropriately.

> *Hello, Ms Oliver. I understand you asked for an urgent appointment. How can I help?*
>
> *It is fortunate that you remembered my warning about pregnancy and lithium. Let's see how we can best help you. Perhaps I can start by reviewing what we already know of your illness over these last few years?*

Introduction   A   B   C   D   E

Use of language   A   B   C   D   E

Establishes rapport   A   B   C   D   E

Establishes agenda   A   B   C   D   E

⌘ Reviews the patient's history based on history given:

> *In summary, it appears that for the first few years of your illness, you had several admissions to hospital, with catastrophic consequences to your personal and work life. However, since starting on lithium therapy two years ago, your mood has stabilized and you have not needed hospitalisation.*

⌘ Briefly confirms that previous episodes of illness involved serious risks to self or others:

> *I understand from your notes that when you have been unwell, it was felt that you were at serious risk of attempting suicide and that you have needed to be detained against your will. This gives me some idea of the seriousness of your previous episodes of illness.*

⌘ Checks patient's view on her illness, its consequences and the benefits she has gained from being on lithium.

Overview of illness   A   B   C   D   E

Confirms risk history   A   B   C   D   E

Usefulness of medication   A   B   C   D   E

⌘ Explains in some detail why there are concerns with pregnancy and lithium:

> *You may recall that when we first started you on Lithium, we said that there were several side-effects it could have, including affecting the kidneys and*

thyroid gland. We explained that regular blood tests would help to ensure that we caught any of these adverse effects early, so that we could take appropriate action. One of the other possible effects is on the unborn child. Therapy with lithium can increase the risk of a malformation of a valve in the baby's heart by twenty times, from one in twenty thousand babies to one in a thousand. This heart defect is called 'Ebstein's anomaly'. The baby is thought to be most at risk between two and six weeks after conception, which is very early on in the pregnancy, and usually even before you know you pregnant. Also there is an increased risk of the baby's thyroid gland being affected, just like your own could be.

⌘ Explains the other risks to be considered:

On the other hand, the other risk to be looked at is what might happen if you stopped the lithium. The main risk is of a relapse of your illness. Research has shown that there is a 50% chance of having a relapse of your illness if lithium is stopped during pregnancy. So, we usually warn people who are on lithium to tell us in advance of when they would like to try to become pregnant, so that we can jointly plan further management. It is thought that the best thing to do is to stop lithium before conception, and to restart it after the first trimester is over, if necessary.

Explores known risks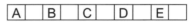

⌘ Explains all options in the current scenario:

In your case we must now look at how to deal with these issues some weeks into the pregnancy.

There are two options at this stage. Firstly, if you feel the risk to your unborn child is more important than the risk to your own health and state of mind, then you might consider stopping the lithium. If so, I would advise that we stop immediately, and monitor you closely in the outpatient clinic until the end of the first trimester, which is the period of highest risk to your child. We can then have a think again about whether you want to restart it from the third trimester onwards. Or, if you prefer, we can avoid it altogether during pregnancy. However, the risk of a relapse is high after the birth, and in case you needed to restart it then, you should not breast feed, in view of the risks of harm to your child.

The next option is to continue the lithium therapy, and this decision might be strengthened from knowing about the potential consequences of your becoming ill again. In view of the risks of Ebstein's anomaly, it is recommended that a more detailed ultrasound scan of the structure of the baby's heart (level 2, 'high resolution') and an echocardiogram (a scan of the functioning of the heart and blood flowing through it) should be done at six weeks and eighteen weeks of pregnancy. In the third trimester, because of the changes in your body, we would have to keep an even closer eye on the levels of lithium in your body by taking more frequent blood samples and we might need to give you higher doses. The dose should drop back to usual levels once the baby is born. Your obstetrician will be closely liaising with us from now on, and they will be watching for thyroid and heart beat problems in the newborn child. Soon after the child is born, we would suggest that you restart lithium again, because of the risk of relapse. I know this is a lot of information to take in all at once, but I will give you a leaflet at the end of this interview which should go over what I have said. Do read through it, discuss it with your partner or other relatives, and hopefully you will be able to make an informed decision. Once you have made a decision, I will inform your GP and your obstetrician. Do you have any questions at this stage?

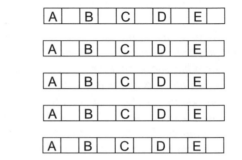

Explains options	A	B	C	D	E
Clear simple terms	A	B	C	D	E
Addresses concerns	A	B	C	D	E
Ending	A	B	C	D	E
Global rating	A	B	C	D	E

44. Discharge plans

There are obviously two issues in this question. Firstly, the discussion with the patient about the discharge plans. Secondly, and more crucially, is the discussion about returning to work.

Introduction.
Confirms the reason for the interview is to discuss after care arrangements.
Also states that they will have discuss the issue of getting back to work.

| Introduction | A | B | C | D | E |

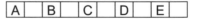

⌘ Explains the written CPA plans

- Outpatient follow-up by SHO at the community mental healthcare team (CMHT) base :

   This means that you will have regular reviews of how you are doing in the psychiatric outpatient clinic. Any changes in medication or other help will be dealt with here. These appointments will be at the community mental health team base, which is not far from where you live. We will let you know in advance of appointments.

- Regular mental health reviews by CPN:

This means you will also have appointments with a CPN. You may recall seeing him at the large meeting. You can talk to him about any concerns you may have or any problems you may be experiencing. These meetings will be at home, though you can arrange to meet elsewhere.

- Continue on depot fluphenazine decanoate 100mg im two-weekly, to be administered at depot clinic.

Your injection will continue to be administered by your community psychiatric nurse, though this will be at the depot clinic at your GP's surgery.

- Patient has contact number for the crisis team:

Should you feel the need to talk to anyone for help in a crisis, you can call this number. It is staffed by experienced staff members like your CPN or social workers and they will alert us if we need to see you earlier in the clinic.

- Next CPA meeting 14 April:

The large meeting you attended is part of the formal process that we have to conduct for all our patients called the 'care programme approach' (CPA). The purpose of these meetings is to gather together all the professionals involved in your care to help plan your discharge back into the community and to ensure you have adequate levels of support and follow-up. As you have suffered a serious breakdown in your mental health, have complex needs, and have more than just one mental health professional involved in your care, we will need to continue to have these meetings regularly. The next such meeting will be on the 14th of April. You can invite anyone else to the meeting if you wish.

- Enhanced level CPA, CPN will be care co-ordinator:

As part of the CPA process, we have to identify all patients who need a higher degree of input from the team, ie. more than one health professional's input. This means that you will be on the 'enhanced level' of care. As there are so many different aspects to deal with, there is usually one person who is allocated the task of being the 'care co-ordinator'. In your case this will be your CPN.

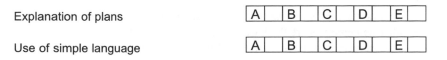

Explanation of plans	A		B		C		D		E	
Use of simple language	A		B		C		D		E	

⌘ Discusses getting back to work:

- The main piece of information you need to keep in mind is that he is a bus driver, and therefore drives a public service vehicle (this constitutes Group 2 entitlement within the guidance of the Driver Vehicle Licensing Agency [DVLA]). He therefore automatically faces a revocation of his driving licence for 'at least three years'. This decision will, of course, be regularly reviewed, as will the medication he is on. He may be permitted to drive again if 'medication is minimal and does not interfere with driving ability and there is no significant likelihood of relapse.'
- Also it is the absolute duty of the treating doctor to inform the DVLA if the patient doesn't understand this advice or drives contrary to that advice (Morgan, 1998).
- Address any concerns or questions the patient may have.

Explains DVLA regulations |A| |B| |C| |D| |E| |

Explains duties of treating doctor |A| |B| |C| |D| |E| |

Addresses patient's concerns |A| |B| |C| |D| |E| |

Ending |A| |B| |C| |D| |E| |

Global rating |A| |B| |C| |D| |E| |

45. Compliance

Introduces self.
Establishes rapport.
Helps to create an environment in which patient can admit to non-compliance.

Introduction |A| |B| |C| |D| |E| |

Communication skills |A| |B| |C| |D| |E| |

⌘ Explores patient's own cognitive representation of his illness:

- this allows you to get an idea of his ideas, misconceptions, and viewpoint of the illness
- a useful way of exploring his concept of the illness is to look at the elements of the 'health beliefs model' (Becker and Maimon, 1975). This looks at:

    ~ what he perceives are the benefits of adherence to treatment
    ~ what he perceives are the barriers to being adherent
    ~ what he perceives is his susceptibility to the illness in future
    ~ what he thinks the severity of the negative consequences will be

- it is also important to have an idea of the patient's perceptions of the threat of illness, benefits and barriers to treatment, relevant modifying factors (such as personality attributes, and the influence of others), and any cues that may prompt the patient to take his medication.

Initial exploration of non-compliance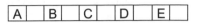

⌘ Identifies whether the non-adherence to treatment is unintentional or intentional:

- intentional non-compliers respond better to more cognitively-oriented interventions.

Distinguishing intentional and
unintentional non-compliance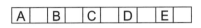

⌘ Discusses cognitive approaches to the intentional non-compliance described (Scott, 1999) These can include:

- using a cost-benefit approach to draw up a table listing the advantages and disadvantages of taking as well as not taking medication. This should then be reflected back to the patient, keeping in mind his current and future aims.
- realistic reappraisals of the illness
- developing a plan to deal with high-risk situations
- trying to address and modify underlying beliefs
- offering the patient greater autonomy via self-management of medication.

Discusses cognitive approaches | A | B | C | D | E |

⌘ Discusses behavioural interventions that may also help:

- simplifying the treatment regime
- using prompts such as notes to self or pairing taking tablets with a routine daily activity
- reinforcement from carers.
- rehearsal of coping strategies to deal with new situations
- keeping a medication diary.

⌘ Addresses any concerns of questions the patient may have

Discusses behavioural interventions | A | B | C | D | E |

Addresses patient's concerns | A | B | C | D | E |

Ending | A | B | C | D | E |

Global rating | A | B | C | D | E |

References

Baldessarini *et al* (1996) Effects of the rate of discontinuing lithium maintenance treatment in bipolar disorders. *J Clin Psychiatry* **57**(10): 441–8. The risk of relapse is higher if lithium is stopped abruptly, ie. over less than fourteen days. Fifty per cent relapse within four months, and 100% over three and a half years of an acute episode

Bauer M (1994) Refractoriness induced by lithium discontinuation despite adequate serum lithium levels. *Am J Psychiatry* **151**(10): 1522. Lithium discontinuation in stable patients, despite adequate lithium levels, has ben reported to induce a refractory state

Becker MH, Maimon LA (1975) Sociobehavioural determinants of compliance with health and medical care recommendations. *Medical Care* **13**: 10–24

Driver Vehicle Licensing Agency guidelines on illness and ability to hold a driving licence. Online at: *www.dvla.gov.uk*

Morgan JF (1998) DVLA and GMC guidelines on 'fitness to drive' and psychiatric disorders: knowledge following an educational campaign. *Med Sci law* **38**: 28–31

National Institute for Clinical Excellence (2002) *Schizophrenia, core interventions in the treatment and management of schizophrenia in primary and secondary care.* NICE guidelines, London

Scott J (1999) Cognitive and behavioural approaches to medication adherence. *Adv Psychiatric Treatment* **8**: 338–47

Useful resources

Baldessarini, RJ, Tondo L, Faedda GL, Suppes TR, Floris G, Rudas N (1996), Effects of the rate of discontinuing lithium maintenance treatment in bipolar disorders. *J Clin Psychiatry* **57**(10):441–8

Bauer M, (1994) Refractoriness induced by lithium discontinuation despite adequate serum lithium levels. *Am J Psychiatry* **151**(10): 1522

Cohen R *et al* (1974), Lithium carbonate, haloperidol and irreversible brain damage. *JAMA* **230**: 1283–7

Cohen R (2000) *Presentations of Clinical Psychiatry*. Quay Books, MA Healthcare Limited, Salisbury

Cohen R (2004) *Vignettes for the MRCPsych, second edition*. Quay Books, MA Healthcare Limited, Salisbury

Cox, Glenice, Rampes, Hagen (2003) Adverse effects of khat: a review. *Adv Psychiatric Treatment* **9**: 456–63

Fukuda K, Strauss SE, Hickie IB, Sharpe M, Dobbins JG, Komaroff AL (1994) Chronic fatigue syndrome: a comprehensive approach to its definition and management. *Ann Int Med* **121**: 953–9

Handley A, Monsieurs K, Bossaert L (2001) ERC guidelines for adult basic life support. *Resuscitation* **48**: 199–205. Online at: www.erc.edu

Morgan JF (1998) DVLA and GMC guidelines on 'fitness to drive' and psychiatric disorders: knowledge following an educational campaign. *Med Sci Law* 38: 28–31

National Institute for Clinical Excellence (2002) *NICE Clinical Guidelines, Schizophrenia; Core interventions in the treatment and management of schizophrenia in primary and secondary care*. NICE, London : December

Reimann *et al* (1996) Indomethacin but not aspirin increases plasma lithium ion levels. *Arch Gen Psychiatry* **143**: 882–4

The Royal College of Psychiatrists (1995) *The ECT Handbook. Council Report CR39*. Royal College of psychiatrists, London (currently under revision)

Taylor D *et al* (2003) *The South London and Maudsley NHS Trust 2003 Prescribing Guidelines*. 7th edn. Martin Dunitz, London

Teasdale G, Jennet B (1974) Assessment of coma and impaired consciousness: a practical scale. *Lancet* **13**: 81–3

Internet

DVLA guidelines on illness and ability to hold a driving licence, online at:www.dvla.gov.uk

Department of Health, online at: www.doh.gov.uk

Resuscitation Council UK, Resuscitation Guidelines 2000, online at: www.resus.org.uk

The Royal College of Psychiatrists, online at: www.rcpsych.ac.uk

www.superego-cafe.com

www.trickcyclists.co.uk